The Biochemistry of MIGRAINE

The Biochemistry of MIGRAINE

M. J. Eadie
Department of Clinical
Neurology and Neuropharmacology
University of Queensland
Brisbane, Australia

J. H. Tyrer
Department of Medicine
University of Queensland
Brisbane, Australia

MTP PRESS LIMITED
a member of the KLUWER ACADEMIC PUBLISHERS GROUP
LANCASTER / BOSTON / THE HAGUE / DORDRECHT

Published in the UK and Europe by
MTP Press Limited
Falcon House
Lancaster, England

British Library Cataloguing in Publication Data

Eadie, Mervyn J.
The biochemistry of migraine.
1. Migraine 2. Biological chemistry
I. Title II. Tyrer, John H.
616.8′5707 RC392

ISBN 0-85200-731-0

Published in the USA by
MTP Press
A division of Kluwer Boston Inc
190 Old Derby Street
Hingham, MA 02043, USA

Library of Congress Cataloging in Publication Data

Eadie, Mervyn J.
The biochemistry of migraine.

Includes bibliographies and index.
1. Migraine. 2. Brain chemistry. I. Tyrer, John H.
II. Title. [DNLM: 1. Migraine. WL 344 E11b]
RC392.E24 1985 616.8′57 85-178

ISBN 0-85200-731-0

Phototypeset by Electronic Village Limited (Richmond)
from ASPIC encoded discs
Printed in Great Britain by
Butler & Tanner Limited
Frome and London

Contents

Preface

Migraine is a very common disorder. It produces considerable human misery. In the community it contributes substantially to absenteeism from work and to inefficiency at work and in the home. Although those who diagnose migraine no doubt consider that they know what is meant by the word, there is in fact no generally agreed and satisfactory brief definition of migraine, and the mechanisms of the disorder continue to be controversial.

A considerable amount of information is now available concerning biochemical changes which occur in man during, and around the time of, migraine attacks. A good deal of this information appears, at least up to a point, internally cohesive. The available data point to disturbances of several interrelated mechanisms which, collectively, suffice to explain many, though not all, of the manifestations of migraine. Some of this apparent cohesiveness may be in a sense artefactual, since the biochemical studies which produced the information may have been prompted by the desire to investigate particular hypotheses of migraine pathogenesis. Even so, the importance of migraine, the bulk of the accumulating biochemical material, and the general sense that this material is pointing in relevant directions, suggest that the time may be appropriate for an attempt at a critical evaluation of the data. Such an attempt may hope to set the material into perspective, to lay bare some of its deficiencies, to make possible some sort of synthesis, and to point the way to future directions for research. From these processes one might hope to gain a better understanding of the molecular events underlying migraine, and on this basis to develop new therapeutic prospects.

No theory of migraine pathogenesis is generally and unreservedly accepted. No known ancillary investigation, not even necropsy, can provide positive evidence for the diagnosis of migraine. In our present state of knowledge the diagnosis of the disorder is of necessity an entirely clinical one. Therefore the clinical phenomena of migraine must serve as the normative criteria against which one assesses the relevance and importance of the physiological and biochemical changes found in the disorder. Because of this, the present book begins with a short description of the major clinical phenomena of migraine, including the predisposing and precipitating factors for the attacks. These clinical phenomena are then interpreted, as far as seems reasonable, in terms of altered physiological mechanisms. Alterations of function, expressed at an organ and tissue level, are ultimately determined by alterations at a molecular level. Hence the reported biochemical changes in migraine, and the biochemical activities of substances known to influence migraine, are next evaluated and related to the alterations in physiology thought responsible for the various clinical phenomena of migraine. Thus the present book moves through the sequence of (a) clinical phenomena, (b) altered physiology and (c) altered biochemistry to reach a position where a synthesis of the available biochemical material into hypotheses of migraine pathogenesis can be attempted. Then directions for future relevant research may emerge. The book concludes with a chapter on cluster headache, a disorder with certain affinities to migraine, but distinct from it, and with a probable pathogenesis which throws some light on the biochemical background to migraine, yet contrasts with it.

It is hoped that the present book will find a readership among those with some background in natural science, be they those who investigate or treat migraine, or those who suffer from it. The book will have served its purpose if it helps advance the endeavour to understand the basis of a common, troublesome, and relatively neglected condition.

In the production of this book the writers are greatly indebted to Mrs Janet Wickham and Margaret McPherson, who patiently and painstakingly converted the many pages of semi-illegible handwriting into an immaculate typescript, to Mr G. Jurott for photographing the illustrations, and to the publishers and their adviser, Dr J. Marks, for many helpful suggestions.

M.J.E.
J.H.T.

Part A
The Clinical Phenomena of Migraine and Their Mechanisms

1
The clinical phenomena

1.1 THE DEFINITION OF MIGRAINE

No generally satisfactory concise definition of migraine appears to exist. The definition commonly used at present, and in part reproduced below, is really a description of migraine phenomena and, perhaps advisedly, provides few insights into cause, or mechanisms of production of the disorder. This definition states that migraine is: a familial disorder characterised by recurrent attacks of headache widely variable in intensity, frequency and duration. Attacks are commonly unilateral and are usually associated with anorexia, nausea and vomiting. In some cases they are preceded by, or associated with, neurological and mood disturbances. All the above characteristics are not necessarily present in each attack or in each patient[1]. The definition then proceeds to describe the range of subvarieties of migraine embraced by the term. There are other operational definitions of migraine, e.g. those of Thrush[2] and Blau[3]. These definitions have much in common with the version quoted above.

It seems generally accepted that the word 'migraine' has arisen as a corruption of the word 'hemicrania'. There are still some who insist that migraine should not be diagnosed unless headache is unilateral. However, early in the present century Gowers[4] wrote ".......the word 'migraine' is losing its original use – that is, its application to strict 'hemicrania', and is employed as a name for paroxysmal headache in general". The general tendency at present is to not require that migraine be unilateral. However the diagnosis is made with greater security if headache involves one side of the head only.

The typical instance of migraine is easy to diagnose clinically. The manifestations will in considerable measure conform with those set down in the descriptive definition reproduced above. The diagnosis becomes more difficult and more contentious when fewer features embodied in the definition are present in a given patient's headaches. What is the irreducible minimum of those features contained in the definition which will suffice for a diagnosis of migraine? Is a diagnosis of 'migraine without headache' tenable, for example, in someone who on the occasion in question experiences solely a disturbance of visual function but who, on other occasions, has experienced an identical visual disturbance as part of an unarguable migrainous headache. These questions are raised, not because it is necessary to resolve them here but because it is desirable to alert the reader at an early stage to the problem of the diagnostic limits of migraine. Sometimes in the literature on the biochemistry of migraine the basis on which the disorder has been diagnosed is unclear. The reader is then left uncertain as to what migrainous manifestations may have been present in the patients who were studied. It seems reasonable to believe that alterations in physiology and biochemistry underlie the various individual clinical manifestations of migraine. If the nature of the latter is not made explicit in a given study, the relation of clinical manifestations to any alterations in tissue or molecular function described tends to be uncertain. The manifestations of migraine differ greatly from sufferer to sufferer, and within the one sufferer may differ in consecutive attacks, or even change during the one attack. It is therefore unreasonable to expect exactly the same set of biochemical changes to occur in every migraine attack in every patient. There is a greater probability that particular biochemical changes will correlate with individual manifestations of the disorder. However, there may be a common core of biochemical alterations which is essential to the occurrence of migraine.

1.2 VARIETIES OF MIGRAINE

Within the category of migraine, the current tendency[5] is to distinguish the following varieties:

(1) classic (al)
(2) common
(3) hemiplegic } 'complicated migraine',
(4) ophthalmoplegic }

and to set them in nosological juxtaposition to cluster (histamine) headache. This categorisation is close to that adopted by the Ad Hoc Committee on Classification of Headache of the American Neurological Association[6]. The Ad Hoc Committee looked on cluster headache and so-called 'lower half' headache as additional sub-varieties of migraine. However the more modern tendency is to see these disorders as probably having a different pathogenesis from that of migraine, though with substantial affinities to it. In this book we have chosen to regard cluster headache as a separate entity. The final Chapter of the book is devoted to it, as a specific topic, though it is mentioned occasionally in earlier chapters, when it occasionally throws some light on aspects of migraine.

In classical migraine painless sensory experiences (most usually visual) precede the headache. In common migraine there is no distinct premonitory sensory experience prior to the onset of the headache. In the hemiplegic and ophthalmoplegic varieties unilateral paresis and external eye muscle paresis respectively occur in association with (usually prior to) the headache. There may be no absolute distinction between these two varieties of complicated migraine and those instances of classical migraine in which hemisensory prodromes include some hand clumsiness, or minimal doubling of vision. (The term 'hemiplegic' migraine is sometimes used to embrace the hemisensory variety[7]). The clinical features of cluster headache (migrainous neuralgia) are quite characteristic, and were elegantly described by Symonds[8]. Variants of this condition are now known, for example chronic paroxymal hemicrania[9,10], with its peculiar responsivenéss to indomethacin[11].

Recently Lance[12,13], after analysing his own experience of migraine, has produced a somewhat different classification of varieties of the disorder. This new classification merits attention, based as it is on careful analysis of an extensive clinical experience. Lance subdivided migraine as follows:

(i) premonitory migraine
(ii) prodromal migraine
    (a) classic migraine
    (b) protracted prodromal migraine
(iii) migraine equivalent
(iv) non-prodomal migraine
    (a) common migraine
    (b) interposed migraine
(v) complicated migraine

Premonitory migraine refers to headache episodes in which changes in mood or alertness, or autonomic disturbance, may precede the headaches by up to 24 hours. The meaning of classic migraine is as in the Ad Hoc Committee Classification, whereas 'protracted prodromal migraine' refers to variants of classic migraine in which the prodromal neurological disturbance persists into the headache phase. Migraine equivalents are, in effect, migrainous prodromes without ensuing headache. Common migraine has its familiar meaning, whereas 'interposed migraine' refers to those migraine attacks in which a neurological deficit occurs during, rather than before, the headache phase. Complicated migraine refers to attacks of the disorder in which a neurological defect persists after cessation of the headache. Thus Lance's classification defines the temporal relation between the (usually prodromal) neurological disturbance of migraine, and the headache element, in much greater detail than the Ad Hoc Committee's Classification did. In a way, Lance's classification regards the neurological disturbance of migraine, and the headache, as semi-independent variables which may develop to different degrees, and at different stages, in any given migraine attack. Use of Lance's classification, with its implicit correlation with the time course of disturbances of function, in relation to the time pattern of the biochemical changes found in migraine attacks, could offer significant advantages in interpreting the biochemical data. Unfortunately the classification is too recently available for it to have yet been applied in much biochemical or other investigational work on migraine.

If any classification of migraine has been used to define those patients who have had biochemical investigation carried out, it has usually been that of the Ad Hoc Committee. Sometimes there appears to have been a preference for studying patients with classical migraine, because of the greater security of diagnosis in this variety of the disorder, as compared with common migraine. The fact has sometimes been lost sight of that the classification of migraine is a classification of migraine attacks and not of people with migraine. At times in the literature certain investigations have been reported as having been carried out in persons with classical migraine, without it being made explicit that the attacks actually investigated were ones of classical migraine. Failure to define precisely the variety of migraine present in the attack studied may sometimes have obscured a relation between biochemical changes and migrainous manifestations.

1.3 THE RELATION BETWEEN MIGRAINE AND CONTRACTION (OR TENSION) HEADACHE

The term 'tension' headache has become quite ambiguous in its connotations. While 'tension' originally referred to muscle tension, inevitable the word has come to be associated, particularly in the lay mind, with an inference of emotional tension. Since emotional tension commonly precipitates migraine attacks, there has developed some tendency to equate migraine, particularly its non-classical varieties, with 'tension' headache. Use of the term 'contraction' headache for the headache entity originally considered due to muscle tension, abandoning the term 'tension' headache altogether, would avoid the ambiguity referred to above, even though 'tension headache' is a concept enshrined in contemporary popular usage.

However, even if only the term contraction headache is used, there remains considerable difficulty in defining where migraine ends and contraction headache begins. An increasing amount of contemporary opinion sees there being virtually a continuum between certain patterns of migraine and contraction headache[14]. In fact this continuity was already acknowledged in the Ad Hoc Committee's Classification of Headache[6], where an entity 'mixed' headache was designated to embrace the situation of those suffering the admixture of migraine and contraction headache.

Sufferers from mixed headache commonly give a history of months or years of episodic headache with migrainous features before they begin to develop continuous headache. This headache has many or all of the features of contraction headache, though there may be intermittent exacerbations which have migrainous characteristics. The head pain in the later phases of individual migraine attacks rather often has many features of contraction headache. Therefore the differentiation between migraine and contraction headache may become difficult, and in the individual attack, and sometimes in the individual sufferer, there may be no sharp boundary. The relevant mechanisms of migraine and contraction headache are discussed later (Chapter 2). Here the intention is merely to make the point that it is sometimes difficult to draw a sharp diagnostic distinction between migraine and contraction headache and that both types of headache may be present simultaneously in the one headache sufferer. In consequence, the policy of using biochemical data from patients with contraction headache as control values for similar data obtained from patients with migraine carries the danger that the control group may contain some persons with the disorder under study as well as with the control disorder.

1.4 THE PREVALENCE OF MIGRAINE

Figures for the estimated prevalence of migraine are highly dependent on how the category 'migraine' is defined and on the zeal with which instances of migraine are sought. A number of studies have suggested that roughly 5% of the population suffer from migraine[15,16]. Kurtzke[17] employed a conservative migraine prevalence of 10% in his recent calculation of the current burden of neurological illness in the United States population. Waters has carried out a series of careful epidemiological field studies in a number of different regions of the United Kingdom[18]. He reported the occurrence of at least one migraine-like headache in the previous 12 months in some 20–30% of the adult populations interviewed. Dalsgaard-Nielsen and Ulrich[19] found a 16% prevalence rate for migraine among Danish doctors, with the figure rising to 23% if 'migraine-like' attacks were included. Goldstein and Chen[20] calculated that approximately 1% of the population each year may become sufferers from disabling headache, including migraine. Bruyn[21] has set out in tabular form published data on the prevalence of migraine.

It is likely that the range of these prevalence figures reflects to a significant extent the way migraine has been diagnosed in the different studies. The present book does not need to concern itself too closely with the true prevalence of the disorder. Even accepting the lower prevalence figures, migraine is patently a very common disorder in the community. If the higher prevalence figures are valid one may have to become concerned at the possibility that a significant number of persons with occasional migraine might happen to be used as normal 'controls' in certain types of migraine study in which restrictive diagnostic criteria for migraine are employed.

1.5 THE CARDINAL CLINICAL FEATURES OF MIGRAINE

To an extent, some of the main clinical features of migraine have already been mentioned in the preceding sections. It is now desirable to amplify those earlier descriptions, which were intended purely to introduce the features which permitted the designation of subvarieties of the disorder. Many descriptions of the clinical features of migraine are available, including statistical analyses of the manifestations in at least two large series, those of Selby and Lance[22] and Olesen[23]. The major clinical features comprise the following.

1.5.1 Headache

While it may be argued, with some justification, that migraine can be manifest in the absence of headache, the diagnosis of such 'migraine equivalents' always seems somewhat uncertain, and incapable of being established unambiguously. Headache is certainly the dominant, if not the essential, manifestation of migraine. The head pain often begins unilaterally, usually in the forehead, temple, occiput or suboccipital region. The pain may remain restricted to its area of commencement throughout the entire course of the attack. Rather more often the pain extends, though not infrequently remaining unilateral, until it covers much or all of the hemicranium: sometimes the pain becomes bilateral, with a restricted or a diffuse distribution: sometimes an initially unilateral and localised pain may migrate to the other side of the head, and on that side also may have a restricted distribution, all during the evolution of a single migraine attack. The pain of migraine remained unilateral in the individual attack in 38% of Selby and Lance's[22] patients, and in 56% of Olesen's[23] cases.

The onset of the headache is usually gradual, the pain taking minutes to hours to achieve its maximum intensity. Rarely the onset is abrupt, with severe pain virtually from the moment of its recognised onset. Not uncommonly the headache begins during sleep, so that the pain may already be severe by the time the sufferer wakens and becomes aware of it. The total duration of the pain in an attack varies considerably from sufferer to sufferer, though on the whole the duration of attacks is reasonably constant for a given individual, at least over a matter of some months. Attacks usually last from 6 to 24 hours; some may be shorter, others may persist for up to several days.

The character of the headache in migraine often changes during the evolution of an attack. In the more severe attacks the pain commonly has a pulsatile, hammering or throbbing character, particularly in the earlier stages and towards the peak of the pain, or when the sufferer undertakes minor exertion. The pain was regarded as pulsatile by 47% of Olesen's[23] series of patients. In some migraineurs the pain never possesses any pulsatile character. The pain of migraine may be a localised boring or burning ache or soreness, particularly in the early stages of an attack. At its peak the character of the pain, if not throbbing in nature, often defeats the sufferer's capacity for description, or confounds his capacity to differentiate between the severity and the character of the sensation. Sometimes the character of the pain of migraine is described in rather extravagant or even lurid terms such as the head being split apart, sensations so unfamiliar to the experience of most hearers as to be rather difficult for them to imagine. As the individual headache progresses, some more perceptive sufferers may note a change in the character of the pain. A commonly encountered description is that the pulsatile element of the pain gradually gives way to a continuous sore 'lifting' ache which is increased by coughing, straining or sudden head movement (contraction headache).

The headache of the migraine attack usually fades away, often disappearing during sleep so that the precise mode of termination of the pain is difficult to define. Occasionally the pain appears to depart over a few minutes. Once therapy is given for an attack the pattern of natural resolution of the pain may be modified by the treatment used.

The severity of the headache in migraine cannot be assessed on any objective basis. Pain by its inherent nature is subjective, and pain that one person regards as severe another may consider mild. Perhaps the most objective basis we have for assessing the severity of the pain of migraine is the extent to which it disrupts the more essential activities of the sufferer's life. Considered on this basis the majority of some sufferers' attacks appear severe, whereas others' are mild; different attacks in the one sufferer often differ in severity.

Commonly the character and severity of a given sufferer's migraine changes gradually over the course of many years. However the pattern may appear stable and consistent over a shorter term , e.g. a few years. Sometimes the sufferer may discern that he has experienced two or more distinct patterns of attack at various stages of his life. At other times the sufferer may be less perceptive, or there may not be a sharp enough distinction between the patterns of the sufferer's various attacks to permit him to define separate varieties of attack occurring in himself.

The frequency with which migraine attacks occur varies widely from sufferer to sufferer. Very rarely status migrainosus (or migranicus) occurs. In this condition repeated attacks of migraine occur so frequently that the sufferer has continuous head pain of dominantly migrainous character, though with an element of contraction headache[24].

1.5.2 Disturbance of neurological function

Temporary disturbances of central (more rarely peripheral) nervous system function occur in many migraine attacks. These neurological disturbances may be manifest prior to the headache (Lance's 'premonitory' and 'prodromal' migraine), or while headache is present ('prolonged' migraine, 'interposed' migraine and 'complicated' migraine). Some of the more common patterns of migraine-associated neurological disturbances are described below. In the experience of Peatfield *et al.*[25], in some 50% of instances the cerebral hemisphere whose dysfunction accounts for the neurological manifestations of migraine is the hemisphere on the side opposite the head pain.

Alterations in mood and higher level neurological function may precede the onset of the headache phase of migraine by as long as 24 hours, and at times even longer. Such changes are usually relatively mild, but appear to be not infrequent. The direction of any mood change is probably more often towards depression than towards euphoria, and there may be corresponding alterations in behaviour. Usually the premonitory mood alteration slowly mounts till the headache begins; thereafter its further course tends to be lost in the discomfort of the headache, and its accompaniments. As well as these probable disturbances of temporal lobe–limbic function, apparent alterations in hypothalamic function may precede the onset of the headache by hours or days. These hypothalamic alterations may be expressed as fluid retention and weight gain, as fever, or as altered desire for food in general, or for particular items of food.

In 'classical' migraine, discrete disturbance of cerebral function precedes the onset of headache, usually by a matter of less than one hour ('prodromal' migraine), but sometimes by many hours ('premonitory' migraine). The neurological defect usually affects vision, as in 41% of Selby and Lance's[22] series. Rarely, vision of only one eye is involved, suggesting that the disturbance has arisen at the level of the retina or optic nerve. Very much more often the pattern of visual affection is highly suggestive of occipital cortical dysfunction. The patterns of the more commonly occurring visual auras of migraine are well known. The disturbance may comprise hallucinatory phenomena which are generally of a relatively simple geometrical pattern and occupy part or all of the fields of vision of both eyes in a distribution compatible with the established effects of visual cortical dysfunction. The pattern of disturbance usually changes as time passes during the aura phase, and may involve 'seeing' flashes of light, coloured mobile balls, migrating 'glow-worms', serrated patterns of brightness, exploding concentric zig-zags and so on. Instead of the positive hallucinations, or sometimes accompanying them, there may be impairment of vision in segments of the visual field – central or paracentral scotomas, peripheral field constriction (tunnel vision), hemianopias. The onset of the visual disturbance is usually fairly abrupt – its pattern commonly changes as the minutes pass – its resolution generally coincides with the onset of the headache. Sometimes there is a brief asymptomatic gap between the two but rather more often the visual disturbance continues into the early headache phase.

Occurring much less commonly than disturbance of vision, though sometimes developing concurrently with it, unilateral somatic sensory alterations may precede the headache of migraine. The sensory changes often begin with tingling or pins and needles in one hand. Over a few minutes the paraesthesiae ascend the forearm and then appear round the angle of the mouth on the same side. Thence they spread to involve the cheek, upper and lower lips (sometimes bilaterally), tongue and roof of the mouth. Less often, the leg and trunk are included in the sensory disturbance. When the sensory disturbance appears to arise from dysfunction of the dominant cerebral hemisphere dysphasic speech disturbance sometimes occurs also. The dysphasia is almost always expressive: disturbance of receptive speech function is quite rare in migraine. Some patients with hemisensory symptoms also complain of ipsilateral weakness, usually of the arm. At times the basis of this complaint appears to be a sensory ataxia rather than true weakness, but degrees of temporary (and occasionally persisting) hemiparesis can undoubtedly occur in these circumstances, e.g. familial hemiplegic migraine[26]. These sensory and motor symptoms rarely last more than half an hour, and usually fade as the headache develops.

Manifestations of brain stem (and sometimes related cranial nerve) disturbance may occur before, and during, migraine headache. Rarely a period of some minutes, or longer, of unequivocal rotational vertigo (not mere vague syncopal dizziness) may usher in the headache of migraine, while during attacks a temporary (or lasting) paralysis of cranial nerve (or cranial nerve nucleus) function may develop , e.g. paresis of oculomotor or facial nerve function (as in so-called basilar artery migraine - ([27-29])). Exceptionally, consciousness is impaired[28].

In the vast majority of instances the neurological disturbances which occur before or during the headache phase of migraine are short-lived, and fully reversible – exceptionally the defects persist ('complicated' migraine[30]).

1.6 DISTURBANCES ACCOMPANYING MIGRAINE

Certain disturbances commonly accompany migraine headaches. Quite possibly many or all of these disturbances are of neurogenic origin though it is conceivable that at least some could involve extraneural mechanisms. Their presence is not necessary to the diagnosis of migraine, though their occurrence adds support to that diagnosis. They are therefore dealt with at this stage, separately from the unarguably neurogenic symptoms of migraine.

Nausea occurs in the majority of migraine attacks, (in 87% [22] or in 86% [23]). Nausea is often accompanied by vomiting (in 56% [22] or in 47% [23]). On the whole, these alimentary disturbances are more frequent in the more severe attacks. Uncommonly they are present from the onset of headache; exceptionally, they precede it. Generally nausea, with vomiting in its wake, develops as the headache mounts, and recedes as the headache lessens. Occasionally, as Latham observed more than a century ago[31], migraine headache resolves rapidly once the sufferer vomits, an experience which leads occasional migraineurs to seek relief by attempting to induce vomiting.

Photophobia, often accompanied by intolerance to noise, is common in migraine, particularly in more severe attacks. Photophobia occurred in 82% of Selby and Lance's[22] series, and photophobia and phonophobia in 49% of Olesen's[23] cases. These symptoms cause many migraine sufferers to seek seclusion, in reduced lighting, during their attacks.

Prostration is another common accompaniment of migraine, particularly the more severe attacks. Whether prostration represents more than the effects of the sum of the consequences of pain, nausea, vomiting, special sensory hyperreactivity and possible neurological defects, is uncertain. A tendency to postural syncope, or more often pre-syncope, is not infrequent during migraine attacks; non-syncopal unconsciousness occurs rarely[28]. Occasionally fever develops during attacks[32].

1.7 FACTORS PREDISPOSING TO MIGRAINE

1.7.1 Inheritance

Roughly 50% of sufferers from migraine give a history of near relatives (parents or siblings) who suffer, or have suffered, from recurrent headaches which appear to be migrainous in nature. Dalsgaard-Nielsen[33] cited a 90% familial incidence of migraine, and Dalsgaard-Nielsen and Ulrich[19] a 61% incidence of a positive family history of the disorder. Nearly a century ago Gowers[34] wrote:

> 'Migraine is strongly hereditary: in more than half the cases inheritance can be traced, and it is usually direct, i.e. other members of the family (very often a parent) suffer from paroxysmal headache'.

When the definition of migraine is not generally agreed, it becomes difficult to determine the exact genetics of the disorder[35]. It is equally difficult to decide whether what is inherited is a tendency to migraine in its own right, or to some factor which itself facilitates migraine. However, any explanation of the biochemical pathogenesis of migraine should take note of the familial tendency to the disorder.

1.7.2 The migrainous personality

It is rather widely believed that certain personality attributes are associated with the tendency to migraine. Such attributes might be inherited. Therefore this association might explain the undoubted familial tendency to migraine referred to above. However, there seems to be little hard evidence that the so-called 'migrainous personality' is a genuine phenomenon. Possibly the conventional image of this personality may reflect the migraineur who can make his (or her) suffering known, rather than the silent majority which endures its migraine more stoically and less vocally.

The popular image of the migraineur is that of the intelligent, sensitive, artistic person of perfectionistic temperament, striving to cope with the demands of life. Yet every clinician must have encountered numerous patients with almost diametrically opposite personality attributes but whose lives are devastated by recurrent migraine. Whether or not the so-called 'migrainous personality' is a genuine phenomenon, it seems clear that such characteristics are not prerequisite for the occurrence of migraine. At the most, these personality traits are likely to be no more than an adjuvant factor to the occurrence of the disorder.

There are other interpretations of the psychological factors underlying migraine such as Crisp's[36] concept that the migraine sufferer lacks the neurotic mechanisms which allow him to defend himself against high levels of affect-laden stimulation.

1.8 FACTORS PRECIPITATING MIGRAINE ATTACKS

Given the tendency to migraine, a number of circumstances seem capable of inducing migraine attacks in predisposed individuals. These circumstances include the following.

1.8.1 Stress and emotion

Migraine attacks become more frequent in many migraineurs at times of stress, and of heightened emotion (67% in Selby and Lance's[22] cases). Sometimes there is a clear and direct relation between particular emotions and individual headaches. Attacks may occur at the peak of the emotion or stress or while the levels of emotion are still rising. Sometimes attacks occur as the stress, or emotion, is resolving, or immediately after it has resolved.

1.8.2 Female sex hormones

In women, migraine commonly occurs premenstrually or at the time of the menses (62% in Selby and Lance's[22] cases). When oral contraceptives had a higher oestrogen content (100 μg) than their present one, use of these preparations was often followed by the development of recurrent migraine after 2 or 3 months. With reduction in the oestrogen content of oral contraceptive tablets this mode of presentation of migraine has become much less frequent. Oestrogen therapy in post-menopausal women is apt to be associated with an increased frequency of migraine, though Nattero[37] reported that headache increased after the menopause in 47% of women. In pregnancy, with its sustained high oestrogen levels, migraine usually becomes much less active.

1.8.3 Foods

Among migraine sufferers and the public more generally there is a widespread notion that particular foods can provoke attacks of migraine. When the evidence in individual patients is examined critically, as by Medina and Diamond[38], the relation between food intake and the occurrence of migraine often appears more a matter of coincidence than of causality. However there are unquestionably individuals in whom intake of particular foodstuffs is consistently associated with the development of migraine. Monro *et al.*[39] found evidence consistent with allergy to particular foods in 2/3 of a group of 47 severe migraineurs, while Egger *et al.*[40] found that an oligoantigenic diet improved migraine in 93% of a group of 88 children who suffered frequent attacks of the disorder. In contrast Selby and Lance[22] noted a relation between food intake and migraine in only 25% of their cases. The more common culprit foods include chocolate, dairy foods, seafoods, citrus fruits and certain meats. Glover *et al.*[41] found that migraine attacks were precipitated by chocolate in 19% of their cases, by cheese in 18% and by citrus fruit in 11%. Hanington[42] has published a list of foods which commonly cause migraine.

Paradoxically, the absence of food intake at the expected time, and also hunger, appear capable of precipitating migraine attacks. Missing a meal, or exercising on an empty stomach, provoked attacks in 7% of a series of cases of migraine[43].

1.8.4 Alcohol

Migraine sufferers often report that alcohol intake appears to induce their attacks. Sometimes alcohol in general appears culpable. More often specific forms of alcohol, notably red wines, are blamed.

1.8.5 Glare

Some migraine sufferers recognise that exposure to glare, or bright light, seems to produce their attacks. This relation was observed in 47% of Selby and Lance's[22] series. Vijayan *et al.*[44] noted that sunlight appeared to activate migraine in 30% of their group of 263 migraineurs.

1.8.6 Fatigue

Physical fatigue, and also lack of sleep, seem to provoke migraine in some sufferers. Curiously, sleeping beyond the individual's usual waking time also appears capable of provoking attacks in a minority of migraine sufferer.

1.8.7 Exertion

Particularly in youth, sustained and severe physical exertion appears able to induce attacks of migraine[45].

1.8.8 Trauma

After a brief interval, minor head injuries insufficient to disturb consciousness may cause migraine in young persons[46]. In so-called 'footballer's migraine'[47] classical migraine may develop within a few minutes of quite minor blows on the head sustained while playing football.

For a factor to be established as a precipitant to migraine in a given individual, there should be a reasonably consistent time relationship between exposure to that factor and the onset of the individual's migraine. When such a criterion is applied, it must be acknowledged that many migraine attacks in many migraine sufferers develop without discernible precipitation (if one refuses to give credence to the unprovable assertion that experienced, but unrecognised, stress may precipitate attacks). It should also be recognised that, in a given individual, factors which consistently precipitate migraine over a number of years may, in the fullness of time, cease to provoke attacks in that individual, though his attacks continue to occur.

1.9 BEHAVIOUR OF THE INDIVIDUAL'S MIGRAINE WITH TIME

Once the disorder begins, the manifestations of migraine in an individual are not immutably fixed for that individual's life-time. Not only may the pattern of his attacks change with time, but within a span of days or weeks he may have individual attacks with quite different clinical features such that these attacks would have to be classified as representing different sub-varities of migraine. Because of this behaviour of migraine in the affected individual, as has already been indicated, when one assesses reported biochemical changes in migraine one should draw a careful distinction between changes reported in those who are prone to migraine, and changes reported in particular migraine attacks (with their individual manifestations and possibly individual peculiar molecular events).

References

1. Editorial Comment (1969). World Federation of Neurology Research Group on Migraine and Headache. *Hemicrania,* **1,** 3–4
2. Thrush, D. (1978). Treatment of Migraine. *British Medical Journal,* **2,** 1004–1005
3. Blau, J.N. (1983). The Definition of Migraine Headache. *Headache,* **23,** 141
4. Gowers, W.R. (1907). *The Borderland of Epilepsy.* London: J. and A. Churchill
5. Dalessio, D.J. (ed.) (1980). *Wolff's Headache and other Head Pain.* New York: Oxford University Press. 4th Edition
6. Ad Hoc Committee on Classification of Headache (1962). Classification of Headache. *Journal of the American Medical Association,* **179,** 717–718
7. Heyck, H. (1972). Varieties of hemiplegic migraine. *Headache,* **12,** 135–142
8. Symonds, C.P. (1956). A particular variety of headache. *Brain,* **79,** 217–232
9. Sjaastad, O. and Dale, I. (1976). A new (?) clinical entity 'chronic paroxysmal hemicrania', 2. *Acta Neurologica Scandinavica,* **54,** 140–159
10. Rapoport, A.M., Sheftell, F.D. and Baskin, S.M. (1981). Chronic paroxysmal hemicrania – case report of the second known definite occurrence in a male. *Cephalalgia,* **1,** 67–69
11. Jensen, N.B., Joensen, P. and Jensen, J. (1982). Chronic paroxysmal hemicrania: continued remission of symptoms and the discontinuation of indomethacin. *Cephalalgia,* **2,** 163–164
12. Lance, J.W. (1981). Headache. *Annals of Neurology,* **10,** 1–10
13. Lance, J.W. (1982). What is migraine? *Advances in Neurology,* **33,** 21–26
14. Saper, J.R. (1982). The mixed headache syndrome: a new presentation. *Headache,* **22,** 284–286
15. Brewis, M., Poskanzer, D.C., Rolland, C. and Miller, H. (1966). Neurological disease in an English city. *Acta Neurologica Scandinavica,* **42,** (Suppl. 24) 1–89
16. Walker, C.H. (1959). Migraine and its relation to hypertension. *British Medical Journal,* **2,** 1430–1433
17. Kurtzke, J.F. (1982). The current neurologic burden of illness and injury in the United States. *Neurology,* **32,** 1207–1214
18. Waters, W.E. (1980). Migraine. In Rose, F.C. (ed.) *Neuroepidemiology.* Tunbridge Wells: Pitman. 384–390.
19. Dalsgaard-Nielsen, T. and Ulrich, J. (1972). Prevalence and heredity of migraine and migrainoid headaches among 461 Danish doctors. *Headache,* **12,** 168–172
20. Goldstein, M. and Chen T.C. (1982). The epidemiology of disabling headache. In Critchley, M., Friedman, A.P., Gorini, S. and Sicuteri, F. (eds.). Headache – Physiopathological and Clinical Concepts. *Advances in Neurology,* **33,** 377–390
21. Bruyn, G.W. (1983). Epidemiology of migraine 'a personal view'. *Headache,* **23,** 127–133
22. Selby, G. and Lance, J.W. (1960). Observations on 500 cases of migraine and allied vascular headache. *Journal of Neurology, Neurosurgery and Psychiatry,* **23,** 23–32
23. Olesen, J. (1978). Some clinical features of the acute migraine attack. An analysis of 750 patients. *Headache,* **18,** 268–271

24. Couch, J.R. and Diamond, S. (1983). Status migrainosus: causative and therapeutic aspects. *Headache,* **23,** 94 – 101
25. Peatfield, R.C., Gawel, M.J. and Rose, F.C. (1981). Asymmetry of the aura and pain in migraine. *Journal of Neurology, Neurosurgery and Psychiatry,* **44,** 846 – 848
26. Jensen, T.S., Voldby, B., Olivarius, B. De F.I. and Jensen F.T. (1981). Cerebral hemodynamics in familial hemiphegic migraine. *Cephalalgia,* **1,** 121 – 125
27. Bickerstaff, E.R. (1961a). Basilar artery migraine. *Lancet,* **1,** 15 – 17
28. Bickerstaff, E.R. (1961b). Impairment of consciousness in migraine. *Lancet,* **1,** 1057 – 1059
29. Swanson, J.W. and Vick, N.A. (1978). Basilar artery migraine: 12 patients, with an attack recorded electroencephalographically. *Neurology,* **28,** 782 – 786
30. Connor, R.C.R. (1961). Complicated migraine. A study of permanent neurological and visual defects caused by migraine. *Lancet,* **2,** 1072 – 1075
31. Latham, P.A. (1872). Clinical lectures on nervous or sick headache. *British Medical Journal,* **1,** 305 – 306; 336 – 337
32. Jacob, J. (1982). Mechanisms of fever occuring in migraine. In Critchley, M., Friedman, P., Gorini, S. and Sicuteri, F. (eds.). Headache – Physiopathological and Clinical Concepts. *Advances in Neurology,* **33,** 127 – 133
33. Dalsgaard-Nielsen, T. (1965). Migraine and heredity. *Acta Neurologica Scandinavica,* **41,** 287 – 300
34. Gowers, W.R. (1893). *A Manual of Disease of the Nervous System.* Vol.2. London: Churchill Livingstone
35. Pratt, R.T.C. (1967). *The Genetics of Neurological Disorder.* London: Oxford University Press
36. Crisp, A.H. (1979). Holistic speculations concerning the origin of migraine. *Trends in Neurosciences,* **2,** 116 – 118
37. Nattero, G. (1982). Menustrual headache. *Advances in Neurology,* **33,** 215 – 226
38. Medina, J.L. and Diamond, S. (1978). The role of diet in migraine. *Headache,* **18,** 31 – 34
39. Monro, J., Brostoff, J., Carini, C. and Zilkha, K.(1980). Food allergy in migraine. Study of dietary exclusion and RAST. *Lancet,* **2,** 1 – 4
40. Egger, J., Carter, X.M., Wilson J., Turner, M.W. and Soothill, J.F. (1983). Is migraine food allergy? A double-blind controlled test of oligoantigenic diet treatment. *Lancet,* **2,** 865 – 869
41. Glover, V., Littlewood, J., Sandler, M., Peatfield, R., Petty, R. and Rose, F.C. (1983). Biochemical predisposition to dietary migraine: the role of phenolsulphotransferase. *Headache,* **23,** 53 – 58
42. Hanington, E. (1980). Diet and migraine. *Journal of Human Nutrition,* **34,** 175 – 180
43. Pearce, J., Ron, M.A. and De Silva, K.L. (1973). Further studies of carbohydrate metabolism in migraine. In Cumings, J.N. (ed.) *Background to Migraine.* London: Heinemann, 28 – 33
44. Vijayan, N., Gould, S. and Watson, C. (1980). Exposure to sun and precipitation of migraine. *Headache,* **20,** 42 – 43
45. Dalessio, D.J. (1974). Effort migraine. *Headache,* **14,** 53
46. Haas, D.C., Pineda, G.S. and Lourie, H. (1975). Juvenile head trauma syndromes and their relationship to migraine. *Archives of Neurology,* **32,** 727 – 730
47. Matthews, W.B. (1972). Footballer's migraine. *British Medical Journal,* **2,** 326 – 327

2

The mechanisms involved in migraine attacks

The clinical phenomena of the migraine attack described in the previous chapter may be seen as comprised of two major elements, the headache and the disturbance of neurological function, together with several elements of lesser magnitude. These two major elements appear to behave to some extent as semi-independent variables in any given attack and in any individual sufferer. The occurrence of headache in one of its varied forms is almost obligatory for the recognition of migraine. The occurrence of neurological disturbance, at least in overt form, is not essential diagnostically. However,such neurological disturbance presents often enough in attacks for any adequate explanation of the mechanism of migraine to need to take it into account, as well as the head pain. While the neurological disturbance, when recognizable, typically precedes the headache, this time sequence is not invariable. Therefore the events which instigate the neurological disturbance, in overt (or perhaps covert) form, may not necessarily be activating factors for the headache. Any adequate account of the mechanism of migraine attacks should at least explain both the neurological disturbance of the disorder and the headache as partly independent phenomena in their mechanisms of production. The other features of migraine such as photophobia, nausea and vomiting nearly always appear to depend on the occurrence of headache in the attacks. These features also require explanation.

2.1 CIRCULATORY ALTERATIONS IN MIGRAINE

Several lines of evidence suggest that alterations in the scalp and the intracranial circulations may account for, or at least contribute to, the major clinical phenomena of migraine. In the discussion that follows we will be at some pains to draw a distinction between intracranial and extracranial circulatory events. At the outset we would point out that, in relation to the intracranial circulation, there are significant differences between the intracerebral and the extracerebral vessels. Extracerebral arteries are under sympathetic control, whereas the intracerebral arteries are mainly under metabolic autoregulatory control[1]. The intracranial vessels also exhibit a blood–brain barrier effect[2]. Some substances are vasoactive elsewhere in the body by virtue of penetrating vascular endothelium before acting in subendothelial structures. These substances may be without effect on intracerebral vessels when they are administered *in vivo* into the circulation itself. However, these same substances may appear active on these same vessels in *ex vivo* situations, particularly if the substances can then penetrate into the walls of these vessels from their adventitial surfaces, as in organ bath tissue studies. Thus results from *in vitro* studies on intra-cerebral vessels may not always be applicable to the *in vivo* situation. It is also worth noting the anatomical point that one major intracranial artery, the middle meningeal, is a branch of the external carotid, and that one extracranial (scalp) artery, the supraorbital, is a terminal branch of the internal carotid. Hence, the terms 'external carotid' and 'extracranial', and 'internal carotid' and 'intracranial', are not completely synonymous in relation to the circulation of the head.

The evidence bearing on cerebral circulatory alterations in migraine derives from both clinical observations and studies using ancillary investigational methods. For convenience of discussion, material which appears more relevant to the headache of migraine will be dealt separately from material which appears more closely related to the neurological deficits which may occur in migraine attacks.

2.1.1 Clinical observations

There are several lines of clinical evidence which are consistent with the possibility that altered cranial vascular activity is related to both the neurological disturbance and the headache of migraine.

2.1.1.1 Headache

The throbbing character of many migraine headaches, with the pulsation occurring in time with the heart beat, suggests that a vascular factor contributes to the pain of migraine. According to Heyck[3] this idea was propounded by Wepfer as long ago as 1727. Some sufferers comment on the presence of distension of scalp vessels (mainly the superficial temporal ones) which they note at the site of their head pain, and they sometimes relate the pain to this vascular distension. The distension of larger scalp vessels can be confirmed by various pulse recording techniques[4]. Particularly in the earlier phase of the attack, digital occlusion of the distended vessels near the hairline, or occlusion of the scalp artery supplying an area of scalp in which migraine headache is experienced, often affords appreciable pain relief while the occlusion is maintained. There is a report[5] that such extracranial vascular occlusion relieves the pain in 37% of migraine attacks, while ipsilateral carotid artery compression in the neck eases the pain in another 30%. However this investigation may not have ensured that patients were always studied only in the early stages of migraine, when benefit from the compression response might be most likely (in other words before any secondary pain producing mechanisms had time to operate – it is pointed out in Section 1.5 that the pain of migraine tends to lose its pulsatile character as the attack evolves, and in Section 1.3 that contraction headache manifestations may appear at later stages of migraine attacks). It should be mentioned that Blau and Dexter[6,7] found that compression of the superficial temporal artery or scalp increased the pain of migraine almost as often as it relieved the pain. Again it is not clear that their cases were studied only in the early stage of attacks. The finding of Drummond and Lance[5] that carotid compression sometimes eased migraine after superficial temporal artery compression had failed suggested to them that there may be an intracranial vascular component to the pain in some cases of migraine. This is contrary to the conclusion that Wolff[4] drew from his studies, but is in keeping with Blau's[8] suggestion that the pain of migraine arises from meningeal vessels, particularly dural venous sinuses. Blau and Dexter[6,7] subsequently argued that their observation that head movement, coughing and straining increased the pain of migraine was in favour of an intracranial origin for the pain. Apparently they did not consider the possibility that these same manoeuvres would increase the pain of any contraction headache element that had developed during the attacks they studied.

The scalp arteries involved in migraine may have an unusual pattern of vascular reactivity between attacks. In the headache-free period in migraineurs Drummond and Lance[9] showed that exercise caused more dilatation of the superficial temporal artery on the side on which headache was usually experienced than on the opposite side.

Whether arterial distension alone is sufficient to cause head pain may be argued. Wolff's[4] experimental investigations suggested that local mechanical distension of the superficial temporal artery was itself capable of causing pain. On the other hand widespread scalp artery dilatation, when it occurs in fever or from the intake of vasodilating agents, does not necessarily produce pain with the character of migraine. However in migraine headache the situation may not be purely that of scalp artery dilation. During attacks the face and forehead are often pale, not red, despite the distended superficial temporal vessels. To explain this Rowbotham and Little[10] suggested that there was dilatation of arteries and veins, but also of arterio-venous anastomoses during migraine attacks, so that scalp capillary flow did not increase. In temporal arteritis there can certainly be severe pain centred on the superficial temporal artery, but the pathogenesis of this pain appears related to arterial wall inflammation rather than to arterial distension and increased amplitude of intraluminal pulsation. Further, the pain of temporal arteritis is not identical to that of migraine. The operation of extra-intracranial artery bypass, carried out to relieve intracranial arterial insufficiency, causes considerable superficial temporal artery distension, but no local headache develops[11]. However, this surgery scarcely leaves the artery and its surrounds intact and operative injury to local peripheral nerves might prevent the experience of pain. In all, it seems likely that, while increased scalp artery pulsation may contribute to the pathogenesis of the pain of migraine, some additional factor is probably involved in the pain production. The nature of two such additional possible factors will be explored at a later stage.

It should again be pointed out that, as the attack of migraine progresses over some hours, the headache often loses its earlier pulsatile character. The pain increasingly takes on a character compatible with muscle contraction (tension) headache, suggesting the development of a changed pain-producing mechanism. The above assessment of vascular factors in the pathogenesis of migraine relates to the earlier phase of the headache mechanism only.

2.1.1.2 The neurological manifestations

Visual changes – The time pattern and spatial distribution of the visual alterations which classically precede the headache of migraine are consistent with a disturbance of function of the visual cortex. The degree and spatial extent of visual cortical disturbance would seem to vary from moment to moment, though the rate of change is nearly always gradually progressive rather than abrupt. Less severe disturbance may cause positive hallucinatory phenomena; more severe disturbance may produce actual loss of vision in segments of the visual fields, or much less often, over the whole of the visual fields. These changes in vision are consistent with the effects of reversible ischaemia of the visual cortex. Bruyn[12] proposed the lateral geniculate body as an alternative site for ischaemia to cause the visual auras of migraine. O'Brien[13] has cited Carroll as reporting that he had seen actual superficial brain artery constriction while carrying out a neurosurgical procedure under local anaesthesia on a patient who had a migraine attack. Vasodilators such as amyl nitrite and carbon dioxide may cause prompt temporary relief of the visual auras of migraine [14].

Sensory and speech alterations – It is convenient to discuss these changes together, as they often occur in the same migrainous attack, if function of the dominant cerebral hemisphere is altered. Whether or not there is a preceding disturbance of vision, the migrainous sensory episode usually follows a relatively stereotyped sequence. At the outset a sensation of numbness and 'pins and needles' appears in one hand and its fingers and over the course of a minute or two extends into the forearm. Then tingling appears around the angle of the mouth on the same side, along the upper and lower lips on that side, on the roof of the mouth and on the tongue. If it is the right side of the body that has been involved expressive speech difficulty often ensues and, very rarely, receptive dysphasia. The trunk and the leg on the affected side are rarely involved by the sensory change. The entire disturbance tends to fade away in 5 – 30 minutes, leaving no residue. The whole course of events is consistent with disturbed function beginning in the most distal portions of the territory of cortical supply of the middle cerebral artery, and spreading proximally to involve more and more of the cortical territory of supply of this vessel. Progressing local spasm or proximo-distal extension of spasm, appears an acceptable explanation for this course of events, and for the almost routine non-involvement of the leg in the disturbance.

Brain stem manifestations – The term 'basilar artery migraine'[15] has been applied to those migraine attacks in which the neurological manifestations involve disturbance of function in what would be interpreted clinically as the basilar artery's territory of supply. Since the posterior cerebral arteries arise from the basilar, it is logical to argue that migraine with visual field disturbance should fall within this rubric. However it is perhaps more conventional usage to require disturbance of brain stem function to occur before the diagnosis of basilar artery migraine is made. Such brain stem disturbances in migraine are not common, and are most usually manifested by vertigo, diplopia and various cranial nerve palsies. On the whole the patterns do not fit with the anatomical site of any single localised lesion. However, the pattern of selective involvement of certain structures does resemble the consequences of the gradients of brain stem neuronal vulnerability to ischaemia that are manifest in organic insufficiency of the posterior intracranial arterial circulation. Thus the effects of differential neuronal vulnerability to ischaemia resulting from reversible vertebro-basilar arterial system spasm appear to be a sufficient explanation for the neurological features of basilar artery migraine. Any type of solitary but reversible lesion progressing by local extension appears less satisfactory as an explanation.

Other neurological manifestations – Other focal neurological disturbances in migraine such as syncope or mood alteration, are either rare, or their anatomical site can not be diagnosed clinically with tolerable certainty. Hence it is difficult to argue from these manifestations to mechanisms involved in their production.

2.1.2 Results of ancillary investigations

2.1.2.1 Headache

Thermography – Infrared sensors have been used to follow scalp temperature changes during migraine attacks[16]. These temperature changes are believed to parallel changes in local cutaneous blood flow. In eight out of twelve migraine attacks skin temperature was found by thermography to be reduced on the side affected by the headache. The fall in skin temperature, in the probable presence of scalp arterial and perhaps venous dilatation, suggests that the dilatation may have stopped at arteriolar level, and not been present in the scalp microcirculation, in which there was probably reduced perfusion. This combination of circulatory events would be possible if there was arterio-venous shunting of blood in the scalp, perhaps with narrowing of precapillary arterioles during migraine attacks.

Scalp venous oxygen concentration measurement – Heyck's[3] measurements of cranial arterio-venous pO_2 differences during migraine attacks showed unusually high blood oxygen contents in the jugular vein draining the side of migraine headache. This finding was interpreted as suggesting that there was increased arterio-venous shunting of blood in the scalp at the site of migraine headache with decreased capillary perfusion of the affected portion of the scalp despite increased blood flow into, and venous blood exit from this area. This interpretation would explain why the headache-affected region of the scalp may be cold during migraine attacks, despite distended feeding arteries and draining veins. (Blau and Dexter[7] noted that facial pallor occurred in 74% of the migraine attacks they studied). It is known that arterio-venous anastomoses do occur in the territory of the external carotid circulation of normal persons, for example in the lips and nasal mucosae[17] and in the dura[10] but the extent to which such anastomoses occur in the scalp itself is not clear.

Scalp blood flow measured by radioactive sodium clearance – Elkind *et al.*[18] used a ^{24}Na clearance measurement technique to demonstrate increased skin blood flow in the fronto-temporal area of the scalp, greater on the affected side, during migraine attacks. Unfortunately it is not certain that this technique yields unambiguous findings.

Conjunctival vessel changes – Ostfeld *et al.*[19] noted arteriolar and venular dilatation in the conjunctiva on the side of the pain in all of a series of 26 migraine sufferers during headache. The conjunctiva appeared hazy and oedematous. Blau and Davis[20] described constriction of the small vessels of the conjunctiva during migraine attacks in six subjects, but dilatation in another five subjects.

Scalp arterial pulse changes – Two or three decades ago a number of studies of scalp arterial pulse characteristics were carried out during migraine attacks. The technical limitations of such studies were pointed out by Brazil and Friedman[21] at the time the work was being done. More reliable methods are now available. The studies did show increased superficial temporal artery pulse amplitudes during migraine attacks[22].

2.1.2.2 The neurological manifestations

Electroencephalography – In clinical neurological practice it is not uncommon to encounter localised or bilateral intermittent (less often continuous) slow activity in the electroencephalograms of patients during migraine attacks, and in the immediate pre-migraine and post-migraine period. Electroencephalograms were abnormal in 29.8% of Selby and Lance's[23] series and in 43% of the series of Smyth and Winter[24] but in only 9.5% of the cases of Lauritzen *et al.*[25]. On the whole the EEG changes tend to be more severe, and to occur more often in persons whose migraine attacks involve the occurrence of neurological abnormalities. However, EEG changes may be absent in persons with very distinct focal neurological deficits during their migraine attacks. Conversely, focal EEG abnormalities may occur in attacks in which there is no clinically evident local or diffuse disturbance in brain functioning.

These localised EEG abnormalities do provide evidence of local alterations in brain functioning during and about the time of at least some migraine attacks, including attacks in which brain dysfunction cannot be detected clinically. However the EEG changes provide no indication of the mechanism underlying the brain disturbance.

Computerised tomography of the head – Computerised tomographic studies of the brains of migraineurs have sometimes shown regional alterations in radiation transmission during attacks, consistent with the presence of local cerebral oedema[26,27]. Studies in the interval between attacks have reported local (often cortical) areas of decreased radiological density suggestive of infarction[26-28].

Because computerised tomography is an expensive investigation that may not always be generally available it is likely that only selected populations of migraineurs have so far been studied with the technique. The selection criterion applied is likely to have often been the suspicion of permanent neurological damage from migraine. Hence such computerised tomographic changes in the brains of migraine sufferers may not be as frequent in the wider community as the current literature reports might suggest. None the less the existence of these changes provides very strong evidence that the neurological disturbances of migraine are of cerebral origin, and suggests that they are due to ischaemia which may sometimes be severe enough to cause cerebral infarction. There are at least two published accounts of fatal cerebral infarction occurring during migraine, both verified by autopsy[29,30].

Angiography – There are several reports in the literature of carotid and vertebral arteriograms being carried out (generally fortuituously) during migraine attacks. Although the published illustrations do not appear very convincing, an angiogram performed during the visual prodrome of a classical migraine attack was claimed to show decreased flow in the internal carotid system with increased filling of the basilar artery[31]. These abnormalities had disappeared when an injection of contrast medium was repeated after the migrainous aura had subsided.

In subsequent reports of carotid angiograms carried out during migraine attacks, the most consistent change has been reflux of contrast medium into the upper end of the basilar artery[32]. This finding suggests the presence of a deceased perfusion pressure in the vertebro-basilar arterial system at the time of the arteriograms. There is one report that this reflux was no longer present when the angiogram was repeated with the patient headache-free. There has also been a report of a vertebral angiogram carried out during a familial hemiplegic migraine attack. The arteriogram showed localised spasm at the upper end of the basilar artery[33]. Such basilar artery spasm could provide an at least provisional explanation for the commonest of the neurological prodromes of migraine, the visual aura. This aura appears to arise from occipital cortical dysfunction and the terminal branches of the basilar artery, the posterior cerebral arteries, provide the blood supply to the occipital cortex.

Doppler blood flow studies – Otis *et al.*[34] and Dalessio[35] described Doppler studies of orbital blood flow which showed abnormalities in nine out of 96 vascular headache sufferers when attack free. The pattern of abnormality was consistent with retrograde arterial flow from the orbit into the intracranial circulation. The findings in these migraineurs were interpreted as providing evidence of vasospasm in the internal carotid circulation persisting in the interval between attacks.

These findings, encountered in a small minority of a series of migraineurs, do provide some indirect evidence for an intracranial circulatory alteration in these persons between attacks of migraine, but they throw no light on what happens during migraine attacks.

Cerebral blood flow studies – There are two main contemporary techniques for measuring cerebral blood flow in man. In one, the radioactive tracer (^{133}Xenon) is injected directly into the internal carotid artery, and the time course of the amount of radiation that is detected by gamma cameras placed over the head provides a measure of ipsilateral regional cerebral blood flow (rCBF). This technique provides no information about vertebro-basilar flow[36]. In the second technique, which is non-invasive, the ^{133}Xe is inhaled. The time course of the intensity of radiation emanating from the head then reflects both intracranial and extracranial blood flow. However the time course of radiation intensity can be decomposed mathematically into two phases; the initial phase of rapid fall in radiation intensity is accepted as being determined by flow in cerebral cortical grey matter[37]. Cerebral blood flow studies need to be interpreted in knowledge of the technique by which the studies were performed, in order to know to what the values of rCBF really refer, viz. cortical flow, or whole hemicranial flow. Recent technical developments, incorporating the use of increased numbers of gamma cameras over the head to detect local radiation emission from more restricted areas, have enhanced the regional specificity of measurement.

The spreading cortical depression of Leão – Work on cerebral blood flow in migraine often makes reference to this phenomenon. The relevant sequence of events belongs to experimental physiology and may not be widely known to clinicians. Therefore a brief account is given here before cerebral blood flow studies in migraine are described.

Spreading depression was first described in 1944 by Leão[38,39], who a year later[40] raised the possibility of its relation to migraine, a matter again suggested by Milner[41]. The phenomenon of spreading depression was reviewed by Marshall[42] and O'Leary and Goldring[43]. More recently some of its biochemical correlates have been defined[44,45]. Spreading depression so far is known to occur only in the experimental situation. It arises in cerebral cortex that is pathological by virtue of circumstances such as exposure to air, to dehydration or to hypoxia. The phenomenon is initiated by various forms of cortical 'injury', e.g. electrical, mechanical, hypoxic, application of KCl. Such 'injuries' may rather inconsistently set up a wave front of suppression of electrical activity of the cortex which spreads over the cerebral surface in all directions from its site of origin at a rate of approximately 3 mm min^{-1}. This rate of spread is similar to the rate at which Lashley[46] calculated ischaemia would have to spread over his own visual cortex to explain a migrainous aura (unaccompanied by headache) that he experienced, an observation that prompted subsequent speculation on the relation between spreading depression and migraine. In spreading depression the decreased responsiveness to evoked cortical activity at a given point lasts 5 – 10 minutes. Sometimes slow waves or spikes occur in place of the depression of electrical activity. It is possible to initiate successive waves of spreading depression by reapplying or continuing to apply the initiating stimulus. Coincident with the depression there is a localised spreading dilatation of pial arteries lasting 1.5 – 3 minutes, with associated increased venous blood flow. Leão[38,39] described an occasional slight prolonged arterial constriction phase following the earlier dilatation. Recently Lauritzen[47] used contemporary techniques to show that, in the rat cerebral cortex, there is a local increase in cerebral blood flow at the onset of the wave of spreading depression, followed by a prolonged decrease in cortical blood flow lasting more than 60 minutes. Biochemically, the appearance of spreading depression is preceeded by increased glycolysis, which occurs before there is a shift of K^+ to brain extracellular fluid. During the phase of increased cerebral blood flow and electrical depression, cortical glucose levels are lowered and there is increased transport of glucose from blood to brain. The molecular mechanisms which cause the depression to develop and spread do not appear to have been determined, though the altered extracellular K^+ concentrations have been suspected of playing a part.

The relevance of these observations to the neurological and vascular phenomena of migraine needs to be considered carefully and critically.

Cerebral blood flow studies in migraine have tended to concentrate on intracranial vascular events, and many of the observations have been made in persons with classical migraine attacks. Indeed, one gets the impression that the act of inserting a needle for angiography or flow studies into the cervical segment of the carotid artery in those predisposed to migraine, or the injection of radiological contrast medium or ^{133}Xe into the lumen of that artery, is capable of provoking an attack of classical (prodromal) migraine[48]. The earlier reports[32,36,49-52] were reasonably consistent in describing decreased cerebral cortical perfusion during the phase of focal neurological deficit in classical migraine attacks. Sometimes the distribution of the decreased rCBF corresponded with the clinical pattern of the neurological dysfunction. On other occasions the area of the decreased rCBF was more extensive than the neurological deficit would have led one to expect[36,51]. Sakai and Meyer[53] found the decreased rCBF was greatest on the side most often affected by headache. In some instances, the deceased rCBF persisted well into the headache phase[52,54], after the clinical neurological deficit had resolved. At this stage increased vascular perfusion of the scalp, or at least increased blood entry into, and exit from the scalp, would be expected (Section 2.1.1). However, in one study, regional cerebral blood flow was increased in 50% of cases during the headache phase[55].

Thus, seemingly in the absence of direct evidence of what was occurring in the extracranial circulation, these cerebral blood flow studies have led to the belief that the migraine mechanism is not simply a sequence of regionally diminished cerebral perfusion (explaining the aura) passing off as enhanced extracranial perfusion (explaining the headache) develops. The flow alterations in the two circulations would appear to behave in greater part as only semi-related variables, a conclusion which could also have been inferred from a careful analysis of the time patterns of the clinical neurological deficits and headache phenomena in a large enough number of migraine attacks. The expectation also developed that common migraine would prove associated with a similar pattern of vascular events, though possibly the reduction in rCBF would be less severe in this variety. However when a group of persons whose migraine had known trigger factors managed to induce attacks of common migraine in themselves – carotid needling seems to provoke classical rather than common migraine – no alteration in rCBF was found during the attacks[56]. This result was used to argue that classical and common migraine are distinct disorders. In a sense this failure to demonstrate altered rCBF in common migraine merely illustrates an extreme case situation of the earlier hypothesis of migraine pathogenesis. Common and classical migraine may both occur in a given individual within a few days of each other. It therefore seems undesirable to have to invoke the presence of two separate disorders in the one person rather than postulate a single disorder in which certain facets of the mechanism can develop to different degrees in different attacks. It should also be pointed out that in each of two cases of spontaneous common migraine he studied Gelmers[57] did demonstrate focal cortical oligaemia, with a patch of hyperaemia, prior to the headache. He appeared to use a similar blood flow measuring apparatus to that employed by Olesen *et al.*[48,56,58].

As the instrumentation for measuring rCBF has been refined, and in particular has achieved greater resolving power, additional information has come to light. In a series of reports initially based on a study of six, but later of nine cases of classical (or hemisensory) migraine, Olesen and his associates[48,54,56,58] have provided evidence that the initial event in such migraine (apparently induced by carotid needling) is a temporary, very localised increase in rCBF, often in the parietal lobe. This is followed by a spreading decrease in rCBF beginning at the occipital pole and extending forward progressively, at a rate of some 2 mm/min^{-1}. It was argued that (i) this mode of progression of oligaemia is not compatible with the consequences of local arterial spasm, (ii) does not correspond in distribution with the territories of the cerebral cortical arterial supply (iii), does not correspond with the pattern of neurological deficit that may be present concurrently, and (iv) would be better explained by the vascular alterations which accompany the so-called spreading depression of Leão. Further it was pointed out that the extent of the decrease in rCBF encountered (mean 36%) usually was not sufficient to produce a degree of ischaemia adequate to disturb brain function (threshold 16–20 ml/100g/min[37]). It is true that the mode and rate of progression of the oligaemia may not be consistent with the effect of static localised segmental arterial spasm. However it may still be be compatible with progressive narrowing of a portion of the cerebral arterial tree. The arguments about the anatomical distribution of the vascular changes appears valid. However, the belief that the vascular changes (spreading oligaemia) resemble those of spreading depression runs contrary to Leão's[38,39] own observation that there is spreading arterial and venous dilatation, only sometimes followed by mild vasoconstriction, in spreading depression. The argument about failure to attain the threshhold of ischaemia necessary to disturb cerebral function may be valid in terms of what applies in persons with structural cerebro-vascular disease (in whom continued oligaemia may have altered cerebral metabolism in favour of increased tolerance to hypoxia). However it is conceivable that a different (higher) threshold for critical oligaemia may apply in the brain which is nearly always normally perfused with arterial blood. Additionally, one should recall that both Skinhoj[32] and Hachinski *et al.*[59] had found a degree of ischaemia which exceeded the threshhold that would cause brain disturbance in their cerebral blood flow studies carried out during attacks of classical migraine. It would therefore seem desirable that all the results of Olesen *et al.* should be confirmed by other workers before they are taken as generally applicable, critically important though they may prove to be. In this connection it should be noted that Gelmers[57], working with what appears to be similar apparatus to that used by Olesen's group, found decreased rCBF in the prodrome phase of spontaneous migraine attacks in two cases. He did not mention the progressing spread of oligaemia described by Olesen *et al.*[58]. It should be pointed out that the ^{133}Xe studies of Olesen and his collaborators were usually preceded by intracarotid injection of angiographic contrast medium. It is conceivable that this prior treatment, or the ^{133}Xe itself, might have been responsible for some of the changes noted by these authors.

It may be worth mentioning that both Simard and Poulson[49] and Sakai and Meyer[50,53] found the decreased rCBF during the migraine prodrome was associated with loss of cerebral vascular autoregulation, so that the normal response of the rCBF to an increased arterial pCO_2 was lost.

2.1.3 Evaluation of the cranial circulatory changes in migraine

There can be little doubt that changes in the scalp and the intracranial circulations occur in an appreciable number of migraine attacks. Further, migraineurs' scalp arteries may show abnormal reactivity to exercise between attacks, and this abnormality is greater on the side usually affected by migraine[59]. Vessels a considerable distance from the site of pain, e.g. the dorsal hand veins, may show heightened reactivity to catecholamines and indoleamines[60]. The autonomic control of the general circulation is altered during migraine attacks, and to a lesser extent between attacks[61]. But to what extent are these circulatory changes, particularly the cranial ones, responsible for the headache of migraine, and for the neurological disturbances of the condition, when these disturbances occur?

2.1.3.1 Headache

The work of Drummond and Lance[5] suggested that extracranial circulatory changes cannot be responsible for producing headache in all attacks of migraine. Intracranial circulatory changes were suggested as an alternative pain-producing mechanism in some cases. However, it is not clear from their publication that Drummond and Lance always studied patients at an early enough stage in individual migraine attacks to be sure that secondary muscle contraction headache had not already become the dominant factor in pain production. Blau[8] had also suggested that the headache in migraine arose from the meningeal vessels. Wolff's[4] classical studies in migraine patients had earlier seemed to exclude the possiblity that the pain arose from distension of intracranial vessels. Despite Wolff's work, unless it can be shown that extracranial vasodilatation occurs at some stage, probably an early one, in the headache phase of every attack of migraine, the hypothesis that migraine headache arises from extracranial vasodilatation becomes untenable. Drummond and Lance's systematic investigation has certainly provided some ground for questioning any continued uncritical acceptance of this hypothesis.

Even if extracranial vasodilatation proves to be invariably present at some stage in migraine, and to coincide in timing and site with the duration and situation of the apparent vascular element of the headache, this does not necessarily mean that the pain is solely due to the vascular changes. The frequently pulsatile character of the pain certainly suggests that the vascular changes play a part in its pathogenesis. However, the argument has been adduced that extracranial vascular dilatation, of itself, is insufficient to cause head pain. Thus strenuous physical exercise, and high fever, which may produce extensive scalp vasodilatation, are not necessarily associated with head pain. Head pain does not occur in relation to the dilated superficial temporal artery that occurs after the operation of extracranial–intracranial arterial bypass[62]. However, it should be emphasised that the pattern of such vasodilatation with its increased skin capillary flow may not be identical with the pattern of scalp vasodilatation in migraine, with its postulated precapillary arteriolar constriction, open arterio-venous shunts and decreased capillary flow[10]. Hence it may still be argued that it is the unique character of the extracranial vascular events of migraine which is, in some way, responsible for pain production. It is also conceivable that there may be some additional local factor, possibly neural or chemical, which must co-exist with the scalp vascular changes of migraine before pain occurs.

At present, probably the best interpretation that can be put on the data is that local scalp vasodilatation, possibly with precapillary arteriolar constriction, at least contributes significantly to the pain of the earlier phase of migraine headache. Other locally-acting factors, possibly neural or chemical, may also have to be involved for pain production to occur. An adequate explanation of the molecular mechanisms of migraine must not only account for the scalp vascular changes, but must show why they may occur in a restricted distribution, and also may change in site even during a single attack of the disorder.

2.1.3.2 Neurological disturbance

For many years temporary focal cerebral ischaemia had appeared a reasonably adequate explanation for the neurological deficits that may occur in migraine. However, during the foregoing account of the intracranial circulatory alterations that have recently been described as occuring in migraine attacks (see p. 24) certain arguments were mentioned, e.g. the absence of a sufficient degree of ischaemia and a lack of correspondence between sites of reduced cerebral perfusion and patterns of neurological disturbance. These arguments call into question the adequacy of the cerebral ischaemia hypothesis in explaining the pathogenesis of brain dysfunction in migraine. It has already been pointed out that these arguments may not be based on unambiguous evidence. One should also recall the observation of Wolff[14] that substances which are thought to act purely as vasodilating agents (i.e. carbon dioxide, amyl nitrite) rapidly but temporarily disperse the visual auras of migraine. In the present state of knowledge local cerebral ischaemia still appears to be the most adequate explanation for the neurological disturbances which may occur in relation to migraine attacks. There seems no necessity to regard the local ischaemia as due to a static localised area of arterial spasm – there may be a changing and more widespread distribution of arterial spasm. A contemporary explanation for the molecular mechanisms of migraine should attempt to account both for the occurrence of such localised cerebral ischaemia, and for its relatively restricted and not necessarily static distribution. In this connection it may be worth mentioning the suggestion that decreased cerebral perfusion in migraine may be a result of decreased brain metabolism, rather than a cause of altered metabolism.

In conjunction with the postulate of a secondary pain mechanism, that of the neck muscle contraction headache mechanism, the vascular hypothesis for the pathogenesis of the headache and neurological features of migraine does go some considerable distance towards accounting for many of the essential phenomena of the disorder. However, observational data to confirm or refute certain aspects of the basis of the hypothesis are not really adequate, and some items of currently available evidence suggest that the hypothesis cannot provide a completely satisfactory explanation for certain experimental findings. Hence alternative mechanisms for the phenomena of migraine have been canvassed by various workers.

2.2 PLATELET CHANGES IN MIGRAINE

In recent times there has been interest in circulating platelet changes during migraine attacks, and in the interval between attacks[63]. The topic has been reviewed by Wachowicz[64] and by Hanington[65-67] who has advanced the hypothesis that migraine is primarily a platelet disorder, with secondary vascular changes. These postulated vascular changes are very much along the lines of those discussed in relation to the vascular hypothesis though they tend not to be set down in detail in Hanington's publications. In light of Hannington's thinking, the platelet alterations in migraine do not provide an alternative to the vascular hypothesis of migraine pathogenesis. Rather they supplement the vascular hypothesis.

In general, there appear to be increased numbers of circulating platelet microaggregates both during migraine attacks and, in migraine sufferers, between attacks[68,69]. Hilton and Cumings[70] noted that migraineurs' platelets were aggregated more readily by serotonin than the platelets from normal persons. Crouch and Hassanein[71] obtained a similar finding, though in relation to ADP-induced aggregation. Masel *et al.*[72] also noted platelet hyperaggragability. In conformity with the earlier reports of Kalendowsky and Austin[73,74] in relation to studies of ADP induced platelet aggregation in persons with complicated migraine, Jones *et al.*[75] found there was increased inducible platelet aggregability in migraine attacks with severe prodromes. This result is quite contrary to the data of Crouch and Hassanein[71], who found no correlation between increased platelet aggregability and neurological deficits in migraine. D'Andrea *et al.*[76] found evidence of platelet activation between migraine attacks (increased circulating levels of β-thromboglobulin and platelet factor 4). The levels of these substances rose further during attacks. Gawel *et al.*[77] had earlier noted increased β-thromboglobulin levels in migraine attacks. Platelet morphology, at electron microscopy, is unaltered in migraineurs[78], and platelet lipid composition does not differ from that of controls according to Bottomley *et al.*[79], though Oxman *et al.*[80] obtained a contrary finding.

A relation between platelets and migraine is also suggested by the observation that in thrombocytopenia (either idiopathic or due to systemic lupus erythematosus) migraine increased when the platelet count fell[81]. Conceivably, increased platelet destruction may release increased quantities of some migraine-producing factor.

The various lines of evidence mentioned above suggest the possibility that platelet changes in migraineurs may contribute to the initiation of the postulated cerebral ischaemia which causes, or at least is a factor in, the production of neurological deficits of migraine. However it is only fair to indicate that the findings of Kalendowsky and Austin[73,74] and Jones *et al.*[75] also raise the possibility that cerebral ischaemic damage in migraine may cause the abnormality of platelet function. Of themselves, the platelet changes could scarcely explain why there should be localised brain ischaemia in migraine. However in migraine if some locally-acting factor decreased regional cerebral perfusion there may be an increased chance that circulating microaggregates would settle out in the slowly perfused microcirculation. This might add a mechanical obstructive element to the functional ischaemia as well as providing a high local concentration of vasoactive substance released from platelets.

It is possible, indeed likely, that the platelet alterations here described may be related to certain of the biochemical abnormalities of migraine, to be discussed in subsequent chapters.

2.3 CENTRAL NERVOUS SYSTEM ALTERATIONS AS A CAUSE OF MIGRAINE

As already indicated, there are certain shortcomings to the vascular hypothesis of the pathogenesis of migraine. As a result, the possibility has been raised that migraine may be primarily and largely the result of a nervous system disturbance.

Sicuteri, whose earlier work had provided a plausible biochemical basis for many aspects of the vascular hypothesis of migraine, appears to have become dissatisfied with the adequacy of this hypothesis by the early 1970s. He then[82-85] developed the idea that the pain of migraine arose because of central nervous system facilitation of incoming pain impulses from the head. Sicuteri's neurally-based hypothesis seemed to derive from his observation that para-chlorophenylalanine, a chemical which depletes brain serotonin levels in animals, produced a generalised sense of hyperalgesia when used in humans for more than a month[86,87]. It also protected against migraine. As far as we are aware, no evidence has ever been provided that there is actual brain serotonin depletion in human migraine (see Section 3.1.2.2). In a variant of Sicuteri's hypothesis, Botney[88] suggested that brain hypoxia, e.g. from basilar artery spasm in the migraine prodrome phase, may deplete brain serotonin and provides the setting for the pain-producing mechanism Sicuteri postulated. This variant of the hypothesis therefore regards the primary disturbance as vascular, the central neural facilitation of pain impulses being a secondary phenomenon. As far as one can discern from his writings, Sicuteri[85,89] did not grapple with the question as to why the postulated brain serotonin depletion augmented the experience of pain in only a local area of the head and sometimes purely on one side. Was this due to a very selective local facilitation of impulses traversing one portion of the central pain pathway? Or was there local peripheral production of pain in the scalp, with a general facilitation and amplification, as it were, of all incoming pain impulses?

Lance and his collaborators have attempted to answer these questions in a way which, in effect, allows a very localised central neural disturbance to both alter cranial vascular reactivity, and also facilitate pain impulse transmission unilaterally in the pain pathway from the head. In brief, Lance[90] and Lance *et al.*[81] suggested that local activation of one locus coeruleus causes noradrenaline-mediated constriction of blood vessels on that side of the head, an effect which appears to be mediated via vasomotor fibres running in the facial nerve. Altered activity of the locus coeruleus may influence descending serotoninergic pathways which connect the nearby mid-brain raphe to (i) the intracerebral vessels[92,93] and (ii) the ipsilateral descending spinal nucleus of the trigeminal[94]. Inhibition of this latter pathway facilitates the transmission of pain impulses across synapses in the spinal trigeminal nucleus[95]. It is suggested that focal inhibition of one locus coeruleus and the nearby raphe could account for the unilateral scalp vasodilatation that occurs in migraine. It would also allow the sensory input from these dilated vessels, with its pulsatile element, to be selectively amplified in the spinal trigeminal nucleus and thus produce the experience of hemicranial pulsatile pain.

Such a hypothesis certainly accounts for many of the cardinal features of migraine headache. Further, if there were earlier neurally-induced constriction of the pial circulation (which could be induced by activation of the locus coeruleus) the hypothesis could also explain the occurrence of temporary cerebral dysfunction in migraine. Migraine might then be seen as primarily neurogenic[96] – something resembling a focal inhibitory epilepsy arising in one locus coeruleus and the nearby midbrain raphe, at times with an initial excitatory phase. The crucial item of evidence to make or break this hypothesis viz. the knowledge that such a localised disturbance does occur in the locus coeruleus, midbrain raphe and spinal trigeminal nucleus during human migraine attacks, is as yet totally lacking. So far, all one knows is that the appropriate neuroanatomical pathways appear to exist[94], but not that they malfunction in migraine, let alone what mechanisms induce their postulated malfunctioning. Furthermore, there is no analogous situation as yet established in human medicine in which a malfunction of the central pain pathway can produce quite localised persisting pain (as distinct from paroxysmal pain). Lesions of the central pain pathway (e.g. the thalamic syndrome, the residue of lateral medullary infarction) produce ill-localised, diffuse, peculiarly distressing pain over much, or all, of half of the body and head. The neural hypothesis of migraine pathogenesis would have to allow the occurrence of a very localised disturbance within one locus coeruleus and the ipsilateral spinal trigeminal nucleus to explain the sometimes very restricted site of head pain in migraine. Moreover, this localised disturbance would also need to be capable of migrating within the locus coeruleus and raphe to explain how the site of the pain of migraine may shift during the one migraine attack. As well, the locus coeruleus and raphe disturbance would also have to be capable of migrating to the locus and raphe on the opposite side to explain those instances of migraine in which the pain transfers from one side of the head to the other as the attack progresses. Additionally, since different migraine attacks in the one individual may begin on different sides of the head, the disturbance could not always begin in the same locus coeruleus-midbrain raphe complex. This inconstancy of site of origin is very different from the situation which applies in partial epilepsy, where the disturbances appear to originate consistently in the one site.

The neural hypothesis of migraine discussed above is ingenious and enticing. Time may prove it, or some refinement of it, valid. However, at the time of writing, unlike the vascular hypothesis, the neural hypothesis has no basis founded on appropriate experimental observations made during attacks of migraine in man. This is its great deficiency.

2.4 HEAD AND NECK MUSCULAR CHANGES IN MIGRAINE

2.4.1 Clinical data

As has been mentioned earlier, in more prolonged attacks of migraine there is sometimes a change in the character of the headache as the attack progresses.

The earlier pubatile headache merges into a sense of generalised tight squeezing head pain which is made momentarily worse by coughing, straining or sudden head movement. This latter pain in its own right appears to have the character of neck muscle 'contraction' headache. If the patient is examined at this late stage in a migraine attack the muscles of the back of his neck – the trapezius and the deeper muscles – feel tight to palpation and are tender to pressure. If the pain is dominantly unilateral the muscle tenderness and tightness is greater on the more painful side. The neck muscle contraction appears to arise as a neurally-mediated reaction to the earlier head pain of apparent vascular origin[21] and there is electromyographic evidence of greater muscle activity on this side (according to Boquet *et al.*[97]). Olesen[98] found such posterior neck muscle tenderness in 69% of the 750 migraine attacks that he studied. Tfelt-Hansen *et al.*[99] noted it in all 50 of a group of cases of common migraine during their attacks. In these patients appropriately placed injections of local anaesthetic eased the pain.

It is also noticeable that when the initial pain of migraine attacks occurs more posteriorly in the head (even in classical migraine, where there can be little question as to the correctness of diagnosis), the throbbing vascular element of the pain tends to be less prominent and the muscle contraction pattern tends to develop earlier and to dominate the clinical picture throughout.

2.4.2 Ancillary investigations

Despite the accessibility of the neck muscles to physical examination relatively little seems to have been published on the use of ancillary investigational techniques, e.g. electromyography, in evaluating the behaviour of the neck muscles during migraine. The investigations of Boquet *et al.*[97] are mentioned above (Section 2.4.1).

2.4.3 Evaluation of the muscle changes

It is believed that sustained contraction of the posterior neck muscles can cause pain in the head, in part by exerting traction on the epicranial aponeurosis. Possibly compression of the greater occipital nerves by the contracted semispinalis capitis may add a neuralgic element to the total amount of pain experienced. It is also possible that sustained muscle contraction produces ischaemic pain within the contracting muscle[100-102]. However Onel *et al.*[103] found evidence of increased blood flow in the splenius capitis during episodic contraction headache. Myers and McCall[11] have shown that experimentally-produced temporalis muscle ischaemia can produce head pain in man. The neck muscle contraction seems to be neurally mediated, and the neural mechanism is presumably activated in the case of migraine by the vascular pain elsewhere in the head. As far as the authors are aware, the exact nature of neural pathways involved in the postulated mechanism remains unknown. However it is tempting to speculate that pain impulses synapsing in the caudal part of the descending spinal nucleus of the trigeminal may somehow activate neighbouring cervical α- or γ-motoneurons, which provide the efferent innervation for the relevant muscles.

The fact that the vascular headache of migraine appears able to initiate another, different, headache mechanism is a matter of some importance. There have been recent writings arguing that there is a continuous spectrum of headache between episodic classical migraine and typical muscle contraction headache. The suggestion has been made that there is no absolute distinction between the two conditions. Certainly the entity of 'mixed' headache, a combination of contraction headache and migraine occuring in the one individual, was recognised by the Ad Hoc Committee on Classification of Headache[104], but in thinking of such a nosological entity it is necessary not to confuse classification of headache with classification of people who suffer from headache. What begins as a primary migrainous vascular headache may evolve into a secondary muscle contraction headache during what is conventionally considered a single attack of migraine. However it is still possible to maintain a distinction between migraine and contraction headache because two separate and distinct causative mechanisms are involved in what the affected individual would regard as a single headache. Further, the headache contraction mechanism appears to be secondary in relation to the migraine. While work could usefully be done to define the mechanism of contraction headache more exactly, the greater problem is to explain the earlier occurring and more fundamental headache of migraine.

2.5 THE MORE COMMON ASSOCIATED FEATURES OF MIGRAINE

2.5.1 Nausea and vomiting

Radiological investigations[105] and the results of drug absorption studies[106,107] suggest the not infrequent occurrence of upper gastrointestinal stasis during migraine attacks. The mechanism responsible for this stasis is not established. Neither is it certain that this stasis is responsible for the nausea of migraine, nor that, in more extreme degree, it causes vomiting. It is conceivable that the nausea and vomiting of migraine arise primarily as medullary disturbances which are not necessarily part of the same train of events that alters upper gastrointestinal motility in migraine attacks. The altered upper gastrointestinal motility might arise locally in the gut wall or be related to some circulating chemical alteration.

2.5.2 Photophobia

There appears to have been little interest in elucidating the mechanism of the photophobia that occurs so commonly in migraine. It is known that there is conjunctival vessel dilatation and local oedema in migraine attacks[4,19,20]. In other disorders where conjunctival vessels are dilated and the conjunctiva is oedematous (such as conjunctivitis, foreign body in the eye) there is photophobia. Therefore it is possible that photophobia in migraine is, like the headache, related to altered extracranial vascular calibre and flow. However, central neural hyperresponsiveness to a sensory input from the conjunctivae may conceivably play a part.

2.5.3 Sono(phono)phobia

There have been suggestions, though there is to the best of our knowledge no evidence, that the noise intolerance of migraine is an aspect of a general neural hypersensitivity to sensory stimuli during attacks.

2.5.4 Disturbance of fluid and electrolyte regulation

Water retention prior to the attack, with diuresis during or following the headache, is not infrequent in migraine. It is usually accepted that these water and ionic disturbances are due to altered hypothalamic – pituitary function. If this is so, these manifestation may be regarded as further expressions of the central nervous system disturbance that may occur in relation to migraine.

2.6 OVERVIEW OF THE MECHANISMS OF MIGRAINE

When the mechanisms involved in migraine are assessed at the level of altered tissue and organ function it would appear that altered vasomotor behaviour in the cranial circulation can go some substantial distance towards explaining the major manifestations of the disorder, including the neurological disturbance. There is, however, a body of opinion suggesting that a primary central nervous system disturbance could also account for the major manifestations of the disorder.

The various biochemical changes described in migraine attacks and in migraine sufferers are now to be considered. Their significance should be assessed in terms of how adequately these molecular changes account for the known (or postulated) alterations in physiology that produce the manifestations of migraine.

References

1. Harper, A.M., Deshmukh, V.D., Rowan, J.O. and Jennett, W.B. (1972). The influence of sympathetic nervous system activity on cerebral blood flow. *Archives of Neurology,* **27,** 1 – 6
2. Harper, A.M., McCulloch, J., Mackenzie, E.T. and Pickard, J.D. (1977). Migraine and the blood – brain barrier. *Lancet,* **1,** 1034 – 1036
3. Heyck, H. (1970). The importance of arterio-venous shunts in the pathogenesis of migraine. In Cochrane, A.L. (Ed.) *Background to Migraine.* London: Heinemann, 19 – 25
4. Wolff, H.G. (1963). *Headache and Other Head Pain.* New York: Oxford University Press, 2nd edition
5. Drummond, P.D. and Lance, J.W. (1983). Extracranial vascular changes and the source of pain in migraine headache *Annals of Neurology,* **13,** 23 – 37
6. Blau, J.N. and Dexter, S.L. (1981). The site of pain origin during migraine attacks. In Rose, F.C. and Zilkha, K.H. (eds.). *Progress in Migraine Research,* **1,** London: Pitman 13 – 16.

7. Blau, J.N. and Dexter, S.L. (1981). The site of pain origin during migraine attacks. *Cephalalgia,* **1,** 143–147
8. Blau, J.N. (1978). Migraine: a vasomotor instability of the meningeal circulation. *Lancet,* **2,** 1136–1139
9. Drummond, P.D. and Lance, J.W. (1981). Extracranial vascular reactivity in migraine and tension headache. *Cephalalgia,* **1,** 149–155
10. Rowbotham, G.F. and Little, E. (1965). New concepts on the aetiology and vascularization of meningiomata: the mechanism of migraine: The chemical processes of the cerebrospinal fluid and the formation of collections of blood or fluid in the subdural space. *British Journal of Surgery,* **52,** 21–24
11. Myers, D.E. and McCall, W.D. Jr. (1983). Head pain as a result of experimental ischemic exercise of the temporalis muscle. *Headache,* **23,** 113–116
12. Bruyn, G.W. (1982). Cerebral cortex and migraine. In Critchley, M, Friedman, A.P., Gorini, S. and Sicuteri, F. (eds.). Migraine: Physiopsychological and Clinical Aspects. *Advances in Neurology,* **33,** 151–169
13. O'Brien, M.D. (1972). The haemodynamics of migraine – a review. *Headache,* **12,** 160–162
14. Wolff, H.G. (1955). Headache mechanisms. *International Archives of Allergy and Applied Immunology,* **7,** 210–278
15. Bickerstaff, E.R. (1961). Basilar artery migraine. *Lancet,* **1,** 15–17
16. Lance, J.W. and Anthony, M. (1971). Thermographic studies in vascular headache. *Medical Journal of Australia,* **1,** 240–243
17. Saxena, P.R. (1978). Arteriovenous shunting and migraine. *Research and Clinical Studies in Headache,* **6,** 89–102
18. Elkind, A.H., Friedman, A.P. and Grossman, J. (1964). Cutaneous blood flow in vascular headaches of the migraine type. *Neurology,* **14,** 24–30
19. Ostfeld, A.M., Reis, D.J., Goodell, H. and Wolff, H.G. (1955). Headache and hydration. The significance of two varieties of fluid accumulation in patients with vascular headache of the migraine type. *Archives of Internal Medicine,* **96,** 142–152
20. Blau, J.N. and Davis, E. (1970). Small blood-vessels in migraine. *Lancet,* **2,** 740–742
21. Brazil, P. and Friedman, A.P. (1956). Craniovascular studies in headache: a report and analysis of pulse volume tracings. *Neurology,* **6,** 96–102
22. Tunis, M. and Wolff, H.G. (1953). Studies in headache: long term observations of the reactivity of the cranial arteries in subjects with vascular headache of the migraine type. *Archives of Neurology and Psychiatry,* **70,** 551–557
23. Selby, G. and Lance, J.W. (1960). Observations on 500 cases of migraine and allied vascular headache. *Journal of Neurology, Neurosurgery and Psychiatry,* **23,** 23–32
24. Smyth, V.O.G. and Winter, A.L. (1964). The EEG in migraine. *Electroencephalography and Clinical Neurophysiology,* **16,** 194–202
25. Lauritzen, M., Trojaborg, W. and Olesen, J. (1981). EEG during attacks of common and classical migraine. *Cephalalgia,* **1,** 63–66
26. Mathew, N.T., Meyer, J.S., Welch, K.M.A. and Neblett, C.R. (1977). Abnormal CT-scans in migraine. *Headache,* **16,** 272–279
27. Mathew, N.T. (1978). Computerized axial tomography in migraine. In Greene, R. (ed.). *Current Concepts in Migraine Research.* New York: Raven Press, 63–71
28. Cala, L.A. and Mastaglia, F.L. (1976). Computerised axial tomography findings in a group of patients with migrainous headaches. *Proceedings of the Australian Association of Neurologists,* **13,** 34–41
29. Guest, I.A. and Woolf, A.L. (1964). Fatal infarction of brain in migraine. *British Medical Journal,* **1,** 225–226
30. Selby, G. and Fryer, J.A. (1984). Fatal migraine. *Clinical and Experimental Neurology,* **20,** 83–90
31. Dukes, H.T. and Vieth, R.G. (1964). Cerebral arteriography during migraine prodrome and headache. *Neurology,* **14,** 636–639
32. Skinhoj, E. (1973). Hemadynamic studies within the brain during migraine. *Archives of Neurology,* **29,** 95–98
33. Jensen, T.S., Olivarius, B. de F., Kraft, M. and Hansen, H.J. (1981). Familial hemiplegic migraine–A reappraisal and a long-term follow up study. *Cephalalgia,* **1,** 33–41

34. Otis, S.M., Smith, R.A., Kroll, A.D., Kransy, S.E., Seltzer, K.A. and Dalessio, D.J. (1979). Vasospasm and vascular headaches: selective vasoconstriction in the carotid vascular system measured by the Doppler ophthalmic method in migraineurs. *Headache,* **19,** 200–203
35. Dalessio, D.J. (ed.) (1980). *Wolff's Headache and Other Head Pain.* New York: Oxford University Press, 4th edition
36. Edmeads, J. (1977). Cerebral blood flow in migraine. *Headache,* **17,** 148–152
37. Marshall, J. (1978). Cerebral blood flow in migraine. In Greene, R. (ed.) *Current Concepts in Migraine Research.* New York: Raven Press, 131–139
38. Leão, A.A.P. (1944). Pial circulation and spreading depression of activity in the cerebral cortex. *Journal of Physiology,* **7,** 391–396
39. Leão, A.A.P. (1944). Spreading depression of activity in cerebral cortex. *Journal of Neurophysiology,* **7,** 359–390
40. Leão, A.A.P. and Morrison, R.S. (1945). Propagation of spreading cortical depression. *Journal of Neurophysiology,* **8,** 33–45
41. Milner, P.M. (1958). Note on a possible correspondence between the scotomas of migraine and spreading depression of Leão. *Electroencephalography and Clinical Neurophysiology,* **10,** 705
42. Marshall, W.H. (1959). Spreading cortical depression of Leão. *Physiology Reviews,* **39,** 239–279
43. O'Leary, J.L. and Goldring, S. (1959). Changes associated with forebrain excitation processes: d.c. potentials of the cerebral cortex. In Field, J. (ed.) *Neurophysiology. Handbook of Physiology.* Washington: American Physiological Society, Section 1, Volume 1, 315–328
44. Shinohara, M. Dollinger, B., Brown, G., Rapoport, S. and Sokoloff, L. (1979). Changes in local cerebral glucose utilisation during and following recovery from spreading cortical depression. *Science,* **203,** 88–190
45. Gjedde, A., Hansen, A.J. and Quistorff, B. (1981). Blood–brain glucose transfer in spreading depression. *Journal of Neurochemistry,* **37,** 807–812
46. Lashley, K.S. (1941). Patterns of cerebral integration indicated by the scotomas of migraine. *Archives of Neurology and Psychiatry,* **46,** 331–339
47. Lauritzen, M. Jorgensen, M.B., Diemer, N.H., Gjedde, A. and Hansen, A.J. (1982). Persistent oligemia of rat cerebral cortex in the wake of spreading depression. *Annals of Neurology,* **12,** 469–474
48. Olesen, J., Lasuritzen, M., Tfelt-Hansen, P., Henricksen, L. and Larsen, B. (1982). Spreading cerebral oligemia in classical and normal cerebral blood flow in common migraine. *Headache,* **22,** 242–248
49. Simard, D. and Paulson, O.B. (1973). Central vasomotor paralysis during migraine attack. *Archives of Neurology,* **29,** 207–209
50. Sakai, F. and Meyer, J.S. (1978). Regional cerebral hemodynamics during migraine and cluster headache measured by the ^{133}Xe inhalation method. *Headache,* **18,** 122–132
51. Norris, J.W., Hachinsky, V.C. and Cooper, P.W. (1975). Changes in cerebral blood flow during a migraine attack. *British Medical Journal,* **3,** 676–684
52. Jensen, T.S., Voldby, B., Olivarius, B. de F. and Jensen, F.T. (1981). Cerebral hemodynamics in familial hemiplegic migraine. *Cephalalgia,* **1,** 121–125
53. Sakai, F. and Meyer, J.S. (1979). Abnormal cerebrovascular reactivity in patients with migraine and cluster headache. *Headache,* **19,** 257–266
54. Lauritzen, M., Olsen, T.S., Lassen, N.A. and Paulson O.B. (1983). Changes in regional cerebral blood flow during the course of classic migraine attacks. *Annals of Neurology,* **13,** 633–641
55. Henry, P.Y., Vernhiet, J., Orgogozo, J.M. and Caille, J.M. (1978). Cerebral blood flow in migraine and cluster headache. *Research and Clinical Studies in Headache,* **6,** 81–88
56. Olesen, J., Tfelt–Hansen, P., Henricksen, L. and Larsen, B. (1981). The common migraine attack may not be initiated by cerebral ischaemia. *Lancet,* **2,** 438–440
57. Gelmers, H.J. (1982). Common migraine attacks preceeded by focal hyperemia and parietal oligemia in the rCBF pattern. *Cephalalgia,* **2,** 29–32
58. Olesen, J., Larsen, B. and Lauritzen, M. (1981). Focal hyperemia followed by spreading oligemia and impaired activation of rCBF in classic migraine. *Annals of Neurology,* **9,** 344–352
59. Hachinski, V.C., Norris, J.W., Cooper, P.W., Larsen, B. and Lassen, N.A. (1977). Serial rCBF determinations during classic migraine. *Acta Neurologica Scandinavica* (Suppl.), **56,** 198–199

60. Franchi, G., Anselmi, B. and Michelacci, S. (1972). Changes in serotonin and catecholamines vascular reactivity during migraine attack. *Research and Clinical Studies in Headache,* **3,** 304 – 309
61. Steiner, T.J., Smith, F.R. and Rose, F.C. (1981). Vasomotor reactivity in migraine. In Rose, F.C. and Zilkha, K.J. (eds.). *Progress in Migraine Research, 1,* London. Pitman 33 – 40
62. Myers, D.E., Boone, S.C. and Gregg, J.M. (1982). Superficial temporal arterial dilation without headache in extracranial – intracranial bypass patients. *Headache,* **22,** 118 – 121
63. Gawel, M.J. and Rose, F.C. (1982). Platelet function in migraineurs. *Advances in Neurology,* **33,** 237 – 242
64. Wachowicz, B. (1982). Platelet activation: its possible role in the migraine mechanism. *Advances in Neurology,* **33,** 243 – 246
65. Hanington, E.(1978). Migraine, a blood disorder? *Lancet,* **2,** 501 – 503
66. Hannington, E. (1981). Further observations on platelet behaviour in migraine. In Rose, F.C. and Zilkha, K.J. (eds.) *Progress in Migraine Research, 1,* London: Pitman. 80 – 84
67. Hannington, E. (1982). Migraine as a blood disorder: preliminary studies. *Advances in Neurology,* **33,** 253 – 256
68. Jones, R.J., Wachowicz, B., Lush, S. and Amess, J.A.L. (1981). Platelet aggregation studies during the migraine attack cycle, in Rose, F.C. and Zilkha, K.J. (eds.). *Progress in Migraine Research,* **1,** London: Pitman 85 – 88
69. Nattero, G., Bulla, A., Levi, E. and Peyretti, F. (1981). Platelet aggregability and migraine: is their relationship a reality? In Rose, F.C. and Zilkha, K.J. (eds.). *Progress in Migraine Research, 1,* London: Pitman. 69 – 79
70. Hilton, B.P. and Cumings, J.N. (1972). 5-Hydroxytryptamine levels and platelet aggregation responses in subjects with acute migraine headaches. *Journal of Neurology, Neurosurgery and Psychiatry,* **35,** 505 – 509
71. Crouch, J.R. and Hassanein, F.R. (1977). Platelet aggregability in migraine. *Neurology,* **27,** 843 – 848
72. Masel, B.E., Chesson, A.L., Peters, B.H., Levin H.S. and Alperin, J.B. (1980). Platelet antagonists in migraine prophylaxis. A clinical trial using aspirin and dipyridamole. *Headache,* **20,** 13 – 18
73. Kalendowsky, Z. and Austin, J.H. (1977). Changes in blood clotting systems during migraine attacks. *Headache,* **16,** 293 – 312
74. Kalendovsky, Z. and Austin, J.H. (1975). 'Complicated migraine', its association with increased platelet aggregability and abnormal plasma coagulation factors. *Headache,* **15,** 18 – 35
75. Jones, R.J., Forsythe, A.M. and Amess, J.A.L. (1982). Platelet aggregation in migraine patients during the headache- free interval. In Critchley, M., Friedman, A.P., Gorini, S. and Sicuteri, F. (eds.). Headache – Physiopathological and Clinical Concepts. *Advances in Neurology,* **33,** 275 – 278
76. D'Andrea, G., Toldo, M., Cortelazzo, S. and Milone, F.F. (1982). Platelet activity in migraine. *Headache,* **22,** 207 – 212
77. Gawel, M., Burkitt, M. and Rose, F.C. (1979). The platelet release reaction during migraine attacks. *Headache,* **19,** 323 – 327
78. Grammeltvedt, A., Hovig, T. and Sjaastad, O. (1974). Electro microscopy of blood platelets in migraine and cluster headache. *Headache,* **14,** 226 – 230
79. Bottomley, J.M., Hanington, E., Jones, R.L. and Chapman, D. (1982). Platelet lipid composition in human migraine. *Headache,* **22,** 256 – 260
80. Oxman, T.E., Hitzemann, R.J. and Smith, R. (1982). Platelet membrane lipid composition and the frequency of migraine. *Headache,* **22,** 261 – 267
81. Damasio, H. and Beck, D. (1978). Migraine, thrombocytopenia and serotonin metabolism. *Lancet,* **1,** 240 – 242
82. Sicuteri, F. (1972). Headache as a possible expression of deficiency of brain 5-hydroxytryptamine (central denervation supersensitivity). *Headache,* **12,** 69 – 72
83. Sicuteri, F. (1973). The ingestion of serotonin precursors (L-5-hydroxytryptophan and L-tryptophan) improves migraine headache. *Headache,* **13,** 19 – 22
84. Sicuteri, F. (1974). Headache biochemistry and pharmacology. *Archives de Neurobiologica,* **37,** 27 – 59
85. Sicuteri, F. (1976). Migraine, a central biochemical dysnociception. *Headache,* **16,** 145 – 159

86. Sicuteri, F., Anselmi, B. and Fanciullacci, M. (1970). A therapeutic trial in migraine with parachlorophenylalamine, a specific serotonin depletor. *Headache,* **10,** 124–125
87. Sicuteri, F., Anselmi, B. and Fanciullacci, M. (1972). Parachlorophenylalanine, an inhibitor of enteramine (serotonin) synthesis in migraine. *Research and Clinical Studies in Headache,* **3,** 310–314
88. Botney, M. (1981). An inquiry into the genesis of migraine headache. *Headache,* **21,** 179–185
89. Sicuteri, G. (1973). The ingestion of serotonin precursors (L-5-hydroxytryptophan and L-tryptophan) improves migraine headache. *Headache,* **13,** 19–22
90. Lance, J.W. (1982). What is migraine? *Advances in Neurology,* **33,** 21–26
91. Lance, J.W., Lambert, G.A., Goadsby, P.J. and Duckworth, J.W. (1983). Brainstem influences on the cephalic circulation: experimental data from cat and monkey of relevance to the mechanism of migraine. *Headache,* **23,** 258–265
92. De La Torre, J.C., Surgeon, J.W. and Walker, R.H. (1977). Effects of locus coeruleus stimulation on cerebral blood flow in selected brain regions. *Acta Neurologica Scandinavica.* **56** (Suppl.64), 104–105
93. Reinhard, J.F.Jr., Liebmann, J.E., Schlosberg, A.T. and Moskowitz, M.A. (1979). Serotonin neurons project to small blood vessels in the brain. *Science,* **206,** 85–87
94. Basbaum, A.I. and Fields, H.L. (1978). Endogenous pain control mechanisms: review and hypothesis. *Annals of Neurology,* **4,** 451–462
95. Jessell, T.M. (1982). Neurotransmitters and CNS disease. Pain. *Lancet,* **2,** 1084–1088
96. Edmeads, J. (1982). Migraine as a model of neurogenic ischemia. *Headache,* **22,** 287–288
97. Boquet, J., Moore, N. and Boismare, F. (1982). Hemicrania and lateralized cervicoscapular muscular hypertonicity. In Critchley, M., Friedman, A.P., Gorini, S. and Sicuteri, F. (eds.) Headache: Physiopathological and Clinical Concepts. *Advances in Neurology,* **33,** 401–405
98. Olesen, J. (1978). Some clinical features of the acute migraine attack. An analysis of 750 patients. *Headache,* **18,** 268–271
99. Tfelt-Hansen, P., Lous, I. and Olesen, J. (1981). Prevalence and significance of muscle tenderness during common migraine attacks. *Headache,* **21,** 49–54
100. Tunis, M.M. and Wolff, H.G. (1954). Studies on headache: cranial artery vasoconstriction and muscle contraction headache. *Archives of Neurology and Psychiatry,* **21,** 425– 434
101. Ostfield, A.M., Reis, D.J. and Wolff, H.G. (1959). Studies in headache: bulbar conjunctival ischemia and muscle contraction headache. *Archives of Neurology and Psychiatry,* **77,** 113–119
102. Robinson, C.A. (1980). Cervical spondylosis and muscle contraction headaches. In Dalessio, D. J. (ed.). *Wolff's Headache and other Head Pain.* New York: Oxford University Press. 362–380
103. Onel, Y., Friedman, A.P. and Grossman, J. (1961). Muscle blood flow studies in muscle-contraction headache. *Neurology,* **11,** 935–939
104. Ad Hoc Committee on Classification of Headache (1962). Classification of headache. *Journal of the American Medical Association,* **179,** 717–718
105. Kreel, L. (1973). The use of metoclopramide in radiology. *Postgraduate Medical Journal,* **49,** (Suppl. 4) 42–45
106. Volans, G.N. (1975). The effects of metoclopramide on the absorption of effervescent aspirin in migraine. *British Journal of Clinical Pharmacology,* **2,** 57–63
107. Ross-Lee, L.M. Eadie, M.J., Heazlewood, V., Bochner, F. and Tyrer, J.H. (1983). Aspirin pharmacokinetics in migraine. The effect of metoclopramide. *European Journal of Clinical Pharmacology,* **24,** 777–785

Part B
Biochemical Changes Reported in Relation to Migraine

Introduction

No animal model for migraine exists. Therefore biochemical studies in the disorder necessarily have been done in humans. This circumstance has restricted the types of tissues in which biochemical observations can be made; in consequence, the great majority of the work has been carried out on peripheral blood. It would be difficult to justify the removal of other human tissues in migraine sufferers to permit biochemical observations on the material. In particular, direct chemical studies on the central nervous system have been almost completely precluded by ethical considerations. Therefore the biochemical work that has been done in migraine has inevitably provided virtually no direct, and relatively little indirect, support for the hypotheses that relates the mechanisms of migraine to central nervous system disturbances. On the other hand, these considerations of accessibility of material for study have not prevented the demonstration of biochemical alteration in the circulating blood. Such biochemical changes go some distance towards providing a molecular basis for the vascular type of hypotheses of migraine pathogenesis.

The biochemical changes reported in relation to migraine seem to fall into several categories:

(i) changes which appear likely to be an integral part of the migraine mechanism;
(ii) changes which appear probable provoking factors for migraine;
(iii) changes which appear to be consequences of migraine;
(iv) changes whose relation to the migraine mechanism appears uncertain, or speculative.

Such a classification assumes a knowledge of the nature of the 'migraine mechanism'. For operational purposes we have chosen to look on the vascular type of hypothesis of migraine production as the 'migraine mechanism'. We take this position both because this type of hypothesis still seems the most satisfactory one currently available, and because it is virtually impossible to see any direct relationship between the great majority of the described (blood) biochemical changes and the hypotheses which relate migraine dominantly to changes within the neuraxis. However, by adopting at this stage such a classification of the categories of biochemical data we would not wish to appear irrevocably committed to one type of hypothesis of the migraine mechanism. Rather, we simply wish to have a way of subdividing the available biochemical data on some reasonably logical basis, so that it may be handled more easily.

As well as the types of biochemical data mentioned above, information is available about exogenous chemical agents which modify migraine attacks, act as migraine preventives, or provoke migraine attacks. The relation of this chemical information to the migraine mechanism also needs to be examined. When the relevant physiological and biochemical data bearing on migraine have been assembled, examined and, as far as possible, correlated, we would hope to find ourselves in a position to attempt a reassessment of possible migraine mechanisms.

3
Biochemical changes which appear part of the migraine mechanism

If one provisionally accepts the general validity of the vascular type of hypothesis of migraine pathogenesis, at least as a matter of operational convenience, one might seek evidence of changes in vasoactive chemicals as a basis for the intracranial vasoconstriction and extracranial vasodilatation of migraine. Such chemicals include the indolealkylamine serotonin (5-hydroxytryptamine), the catecholamines (principally dopamine, noradrenaline and adrenaline), their synthesising and degradative enzymes, histamine and its degradative enzyme diamine oxidase, certain vasoactive oligopeptides (notably bradykinin) and various eicosanoids (prostaglandins). As it happens, some members of these groups of chemicals also possess pain producing properties.

3.1 SEROTONIN AND RELATED INDOLEALKYLAMINES

3.1.1 Biology

3.1.1.1 Formation

The indolealkylamines are derived from the essential aromatic aminoacid tryptophan (Figure 3.1). Tryptophan is first hydroxylated at the 5 position on the indole ring, in a reaction catalysed by the enzyme tryptophan hydroxylase, to form 5-hydroxytryptophan. Both tryptophan and its 5-hydroxy derivative can be transported across cell membranes, including those which constitute the blood–brain barrier. 5-hydroxytryptophan subsequent undergoes decarboxylation to form 5-hydroxytryptamine (serotonin). This reaction is catalysed by the enzyme aromatic L-aminoacid decarboxylase, which utilises pyridoxal phosphate as a coenzyme. This decarboxylase and the enzyme which catalyses the decarboxylation of the catecholamine precursor tyrosine are often considered identical.

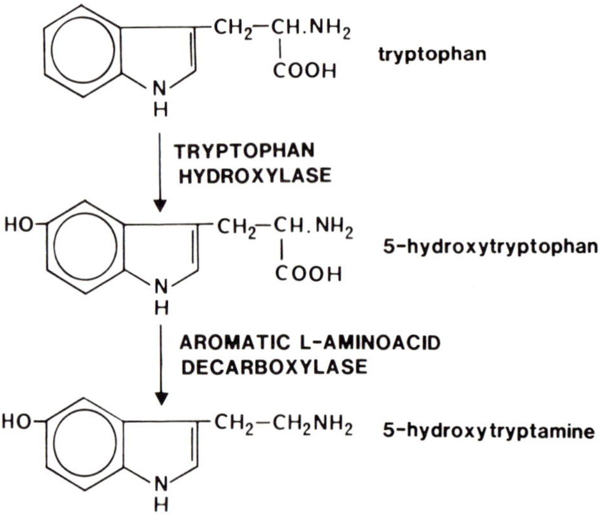

Figure 3.1 Formation of 5-hydroxytryptamine from tryptophan

At most sites in the body 5-hydroxytryptamine represents the final stage of indolealkylamine synthesis, though tryptophan can also be decarboxylated to tryptamine, without 5-hydroxylation at any stage. However, in the pineal, serotonin is further metabolised to certain indolealkylamine conjugates. Two enzymes are involved: *N*-acetyltransferase, which transfers an acetyl group to add to the terminal primary amine moiety of serotonin, and 5-hydroxyindole-*O*-methyl transferase, which transfers a -CH_3 group from *S*-adenosyl methionine to conjugate with the hydroxy group attached to the 5 position of the indole ring. Serotonin may be either *O*-methylated or acetylated as the first conjugation stage, and the *O*-methyl and acetyl conjugates are then acetylated or *O*-methylated respectively to form 5-methoxy-*N*-acetyltryptamine (melatonin) (Figure 3.2).

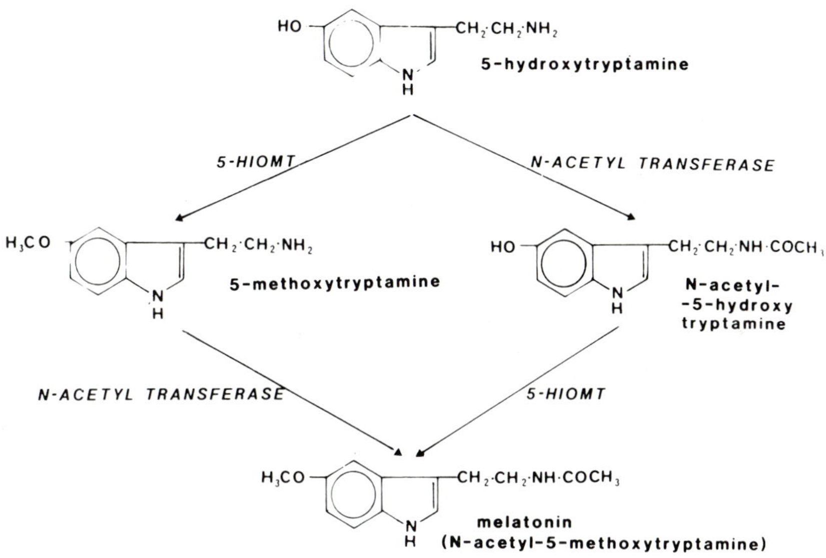

Figure 3.2 Conversion of 5-hydroxytryptamine to melatonin

3.1.1.2 Degradation

The main routes of metabolism of 5-hydroxytryptamine are:

(1) oxidative deamination, catalysed by the mitochondrial enzyme monoamine oxidase;
(2) 5-*O*-methylation and acetylation, described above in relation to melatonin formation, and important only in relation to the pineal

The initial product of monoamine oxidase activity is 5-hydroxyindoleacetaldehyde. This may then be:

(1) further oxidised, in a reaction catalysed by the enzyme aldehyde dehydrogenase, to form 5-hydroxyindoleacetic acid, which appears in urine (partly in conjugated form) as the main metabolite of 5-hydroxytryptamine;
(2) reduced, in a reaction catalysed by aldehyde reductase, to form an alcohol, 5-hydroxy-tryptophol. This may subsequently give rise to an *O*-acetyl

The various 5-hydroxy derivatives of serotonin may undergo *O*-methylation at the 5-position: further, these different 5-methoxy derivatives of 5-hydroxytryptamine may then be oxidised by monoamine oxidase, and the aliphatic acid products may undergo further oxidation, or may be reduced and then *O*-acetylated. The full gamut of known reactions is illustrated by Smith, Francis and Mullen[1]. A selection of the reactions, principally those which at the present time seem most relevant medically, is set out in Figure 3.3.

3.1.1.3 Sites of occurrence in the body

The main sites of occurrence of serotonin and its immediate precursors and derivatives are the brain, the wall of the gastrointestinal tract, and the circulating platelets.

In the brain serotonin occurs in specific regions such as neurons of the mid brain raphe which project (a) rostrally, to the forebrain, then sweep back to reach many parts of the cortex (b) caudally, to synapse on neurons of the substantia gelantinosa of the spinal cord and the analogous neurons of the descending spinal nucleus of the trigeminal nerve. Serotonin also occurs at high concentration, probably higher than anywhere else in the body, in the pineal. Here its concentrations are highest in hours of daylight. Pineal serotonin concentrations fall overnight when, under β-noradrenergic control exercised via sympathetic nerves arising from the superior cervical ganglion, the pinealocytes 'turn on' their *N*-acetyltransferase activity, leading to conversion of serotonin to melatonin. The methoxy derivatives of serotonin in the nervous system occur mainly in the pineal.

In the gastrointestinal tract serotonin is formed and stored in the enterochromaffin cells in the gastric and small intestinal mucosae. Some 90% of body serotonin is said to be present in the alimentary tract. Platelets are believed to lack the enzymes required to synthesise serotonin[2,3] though Lingjaerde[4] stated that human platelets contain sufficient tryptophan hydroxylase activity to form serotonin.

Platelets have active uptake mechanisms for serotonin and store the amine in high concentration in their storage granules (dense bodies). Mean platelet serotonin content is 1.67 nmol/mg of platelet protein[3] or 391.6 ng/10^9 platelets[5]. Platelets also contain considerable amounts of serotonin in the form of sulphate conjugates. After platelets aggregate they release serotonin. They appear to have the capacity to metabolise serotonin slowly to 5-hydroxyindoleacetic acid and 5-hydroxytryptophol[2] and, at least in rabbits, to melatonin[6]. If platelets cannot synthesise serotonin, the question arises: how do they obtain their serotonin content? There appears to be very little serotonin present in platelet-free plasma: some contend that there is none. The difficulty in obtaining a reliable value for plasma water serotonin content lies in the possibility of a few platelets rupturing during their separation from plasma, and thus releasing their serotonin content into plasma, where it may subsequently be measured. However, if no serotonin does occur in platelet-free plasma anywhere in the body, and the platelets lack the enzymatic apparatus necessary for serotonin manufacture, it becomes rather difficult to see how the platelets can acquire their serotonin content. Therefore one is inclined to the view that some serotonin must be present in the platelet-free component of circulating plasma, at least at times, though perhaps mainly in the portal circulation[7]. Even if this is so, the lower of the published figures for platelet poor plasma serotonin (6.5 μg/l (ref.3), 26–38 μg/l(ref.8),25.33 μg/l (ref.5) may still be overestimates of the parameter. Where is the site of origin of plasma and platelet serotonin? The conventional answer, derived more or less by default, is that the origin is in the wall of the gastrointestinal tract. In animals, platelet serotonin almost disappears after extensive resection of the alimentary tract[4]. However, one should remember that the pineal is one of these circumventricular organs which lie outside the blood–brain barrier. One cannot discount the possibility that the pineal may contribute to the serotonin content of circulating plasma and its platelets.

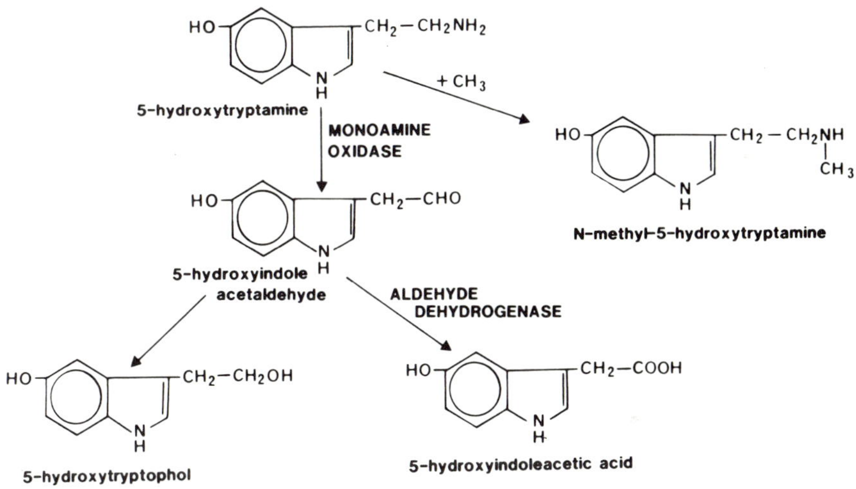

Figure 3.3 Metabolism of 5-hydroxytryptamine

Total plasma serotonin level shows some diurnal fluctuation, but no consistent pattern. Mean values are (males) 0.78, and females 1.0 μg/10^9 platelets.

3.1.1.4 Effects of serotonin

There appear to be at least two types of serotonin receptor in the body[9]. These types are designated $5HT_1(S_1)$and $5HT_2(S_2)$. The $5HT_1$ receptors are linked to adenylate cyclase. Many central nervous and vascular effects of serotonin appear mediated via $5HT_2$ receptors[10]. Some peripheral noradrenergic axon terminals possess prejunctional serotonin receptors which influence noradrenaline release[11]. These M receptors appear to differ from the $5HT_1$ and $5HT_2$ subtypes.

Brain In the nervous system serotonin is an established neurotransmitter. The descending serotoninergic pathways from the midbrain raphe (which contains $5HT_1$ receptors[12]) to the substantia gelatinosa and spinal nucleus of the trigeminal appear to modulate the transmission of pain impulses at synapses between the first and second sensory neurons. Central serotonin depletion appears to facilitate the transmission of pain impulses, and to thus augment the experience of pain. The ascending serotoninergic pathways to the forebrain appear to project widely and to influence the activity of a considerable variety of cortical neurons. Increased central serotonin levels appear to promote sleep, and it is possible that central serotonin depletion may play a causative role in depressive illness.

Peripheral nerve endings At pain-sensitive afferent nerve terminals in the periphery, serotonin appears capable of initiating pain impulses[13]. However,the presence of the oligopeptide bradykinin, and certain eicosanoids (prostaglandins) appears necessary for this effect to occur.

Alimentary tract The relation between serotonin and alimentary tract function was discussed by Thompson[14]. Serotonin applied to the mucosal surface of the gut appears to cause enhanced contractility of the smooth muscle of the gastrointestinal tract, leading to increased peristaltic activity[15,16]. This action is mediated via $5HT_1$ receptors[9]. However, applied to the serosal surface of the gut, serotonin inhibits peristalsis[15,17,18], possibly by acting on ganglion cells which have an inhibitory function.

Circulation The role of serotonin in vascular function has been critically reviewed by Vanhoutte and Cohen[19]. By acting on $5HT_2$ receptors to cause vascular smooth muscle contraction[20], circulating serotonin constricts arteries and veins in many vascular beds[21] including the external carotid system[22]. The venoconstrictor action, particularly on cranial vessels, is a potent one[23]. However serotonin causes vasodilatation in skeletal muscle, and also tends to dilate arterioles, particularly in the splanchnic and cerebral circulations[24].

Edvinsson and MacKenzie[25] reviewed the data available to 1977 relating to the actions of serotonin on the cerebral circulation. In assessing the effects of serotonin on this circulation it may be useful to point out that the amine does not cross the intact blood – brain barrier. Therefore it may not be able to gain access to the muscle coats of intracerebral vessels to exert a vasoconstrictor effect *in vivo*[26], whereas if it is applied to segments of the same vessels in an organ bath there may be no limitation of access. Hence vasoconstriction may occur in such an experimental preparation, yet not *in vivo*. Grimson *et al.*[27] reported that serotonin infused into the baboon internal carotid artery caused decreased blood flow, but if infused into the external carotid caused vasodilatation and increased flow. Deshmukh and Harper[28] also showed that, in baboons, intracarotid serotonin infusion increased external carotid blood flow and scalp muscle blood flow, but decreased internal carotid flow. However, the work of Edvisson and Hardebro[29] produced a result which complicated the issue. They found that intracarotid serotonin administration increased external carotid flow in the baboon, but decreased it in the monkey, an observation raising the question of species specifity of effects. Welch *et al.*[30] and Lance *et al.*[31] found in macaque monkeys that intracarotid serotonin infusion caused a dose-dependent decrease in external (and also internal) carotid blood flow.

However Edvisson and MacKenzie[25] pointed out that intracarotid serotonin administration might disrupt the blood – brain barrier and lead to decreased cerebral blood flow by allowing circulating amines better access to vascular smooth muscles than would apply in more physiological circumstances. Saxena and Tangri[32] reported that serotonin infusion in cats caused decreased flow through cranial arteriovenous shunts.

Edvinsson and Hardebo[29] reported that serotonin contracted previously relaxed segments of human temporal and pial arteries, but relaxed them if their tone had already been raised by prior exposure to prostaglandin $F_{2\alpha}$. Saxena[33] stated that in man serotonin constricts intracranial and extracranial arteries. Burnstock[34] claimed that serotonin dilates cerebral arterioles, but constricts larger arteries. He indicated that intracranial vessels are more responsive to the amine than extracranial ones. Olesen and Skinhoj[35] found that, infused intravenously, serotonin did not alter cerebral blood flow in man to a significant extent. Lance *et al.*[36] infused serotonin into the carotid system of migraineurs and showed that the superficial temporal artery constricted on the side of the infusion. Slight intracranial vasoconstriction also occurred. Olesen[37] carried out intra-arterial ^{133}Xe cerebral blood flow studies in man and showed that an internal carotid infusion of serotonin lasting 2 – 5 minutes produced only a non-statistically significant decrease in regional cerebral blood flow. This finding agreed with the earlier work of Olesen and Skinhoj[35].

It should also be noted that, as well as circulating serotonin affecting blood flow by its effects on vascular musculature, the amine may affect vascular behaviour through neural mechanisms via a network of nerves arising from the raphe and innervating intracerebral blood vessels (see Section 2.3).

Serotonin may cause raised plasma catecholamine levels[38].

Platelets Serotonin, including serotonin released from platelets, acts on $5HT_2$ type receptors to promote platelet aggregation, which leads to further serotonin release. However, serotonin has relatively little effect on human platelets, causing mainly shape change and reversible aggregation[39].

3.1.1.5 Effects of melatonin

The biological role of melatonin in man is still being explored. In plasma its concentrations, which reflect its synthesis by the pineal, undergo a 24-hour cyclical course. Plasma melatonin levels are much higher in darkness than in daylight. Stress appears to have little influence on the circulating levels of the neurohormone. Reduced melatonin levels appear to bear some relationship to depression, and increased levels to mania[40]. It is possible that melatonin function is related in some way to the events of puberty in humans, but there are certain conflicting data. Melatonin in man appears to promote drowsiness, and to have a tranquillising effect.

Melatonin is reported to inhibit platelet aggregability[41].

3.1.1.6 Effects of 5-methoxytryptamine

In vitro 5-methoxytryptamine is reported to be nearly as potent a constrictor of the isolated human basilar artery as is serotonin itself[42].

3.1.1.7 Effects of other indolealkylamines and their derivatives

Whether the other various serotonin metabolites mentioned above are biologically active is as yet unclear. The question has not yet been investigated adequately. The *N*-dimethyl derivatives of tryptamine are known to be psychoactive but it is not yet certain that these substances are of endogenous origin in man, let alone that they play a role in spontaneous human psychiatric disorders.

3.1.2 Serotonin alterations in migraine

3.1.2.1 Circulating serotonin

Sicuteri *et al.*[43] provided the first evidence of possible involvement of serotonin in the biochemical pathogenesis of migraine. They demonstrated increased urinary excretion of the main serotonin metabolite, 5-hydroxyindoleacetic acid, during migraine attacks in 15 subjects. Urine volumes were not stated, and it is therefore possible that the increase in urine 5-hydroxyindoleacetic acid excretion from a mean 4.0 to a mean 10.6 mg/day could represent, in part or in whole, the consequences of diuresis. This finding of increased serotonin metabolite excretion has been confirmed in certain subsequent studies[44-47]. In general, there has been little discussion of the possibility that diuresis might contribute to the increased 5-hydroxyindoleacetic acid excretion. However, Blau *et al.*[48], Curzon *et al.*[49] and Curzon[50] failed to find consistently increased serotonin metabolite excretion in urine during migraine attacks. Kangasniemi *et al.*[51] described increased urinary excretion of unconjugated 5-hydroxyindoleacetic acid in only four out of nine migraineurs during attacks, and decreased excretion in two. Excretion of conjugated serotonin metabolite was increased in five out of six subjects. Nattero[52] reported decreased urinary 5-hydroxyindoleacetic acid excretion in attacks of menstrual migraine. Increased urinary excretion of serotonin itself during migraine attacks was reported by Anthony and Hinterberger[53]. Mück-Šeler *et al.*[47] found a slight, not statistically significant rise in urine serotonin excretion during migraine, with a fall in its excretion after attacks.

Beginning with Curran *et al.*[44], a number of workers have demonstrated reduced total plasma (or platelet rich plasma or platelet) serotonin levels during a substantial majority of the migraine attacks they studied [47,54-62]. Anthony *et al.*[56] obtained evidence that the serotonin change was not simply a non-specific effect of stress or pain.

Sjaastad[63,64] pointed out the need to distinguish between plasma water (or, in practice, platelet-poor plasma) serotonin, and serotonin measured in whole plasma or platelet containing plasma. The serotonin in platelets is not available to influence vascular tone. Somerville[65] reported a mean decrease of 35.8% (from 17.6 to 11.3 ng/ml) in mean platelet-poor plasma serotonin concentration in four subjects during migraine attacks. This appears to be the earliest attempt to measure concentrations of the amine in plasma free of platelets and collected during migraine attacks. Unfortunately, Somerville's values for the parameter are several times greater than those obtained by using contemporary methods for the measurement of serotonin content of platelet-poor plasma. Possibly Somerville's findings are invalid because of unrecognised platelet contamination, or release of serotonin from damaged platelets during separation of cellular elements from plasma prior to measurement of the indolealkylamine. Salmon *et al.*[66] more recently found a mean platelet-poor plasma serotonin level of 18.10 ng/ml during migraine attacks, with a mean level in control subjects of 25.33 ng/ml. There was no change in the levels measured during and between migraine attacks. The same methodology criticisms may apply to this work as to Somerville's[65]. It is also possible that the measurements may not have been made early enough in migraine attacks to detect relevant but temporary plasma water serotonin changes.

Hyppä and Kangasniemi[67] found no change in the plasma level of the serotonin precursor tryptophan in migraine. In direct contrast Salmon *et al.*[68] and Anselmi *et al.*[69] reported increased levels of plasma unbound tryptophan on the day before, the day of and the day after migraine attacks. Cerebrospinal fluid tryptophan levels were found to rise during migraine[68,69].

There is a good deal of evidence that platelet serotonin levels are reduced during migraine attacks, but there is no unambiguous evidence as to what happens to serotonin in platelet-free plasma at the same time. The platelet serotonin changes appear to have occurred in the great majority of reported cases, though these changes have not been invariable; nor have they always been of large magnitude, since they average only about 20% of the value for attack-free platelet (or platelet-rich plasma) serotonin levels. Taken in conjunction with the reports of increased urine 5-hydroxyindoleacetic acid excretion during migraine attacks, this fall in platelet serotonin content has usually been interpreted as suggesting that platelets have released part of their serotonin content during migraine, and that this released serotonin has then been metabolised to 5-hydroxyindoleacetic acid. However, the evidence for the latter sequence is far from conclusive. To put the interpretation on a firmer basis one would wish to know:

(1) that there was a rise in plasma hydroxyindoleacetic acid as well as an increased urinary excretion of this substance, plus its conjugates, during migraine attacks and that these changes followed the fall in platelet serotonin content; and
(2) that serial measurements of platelet and plasma water serotonin throughout migraine attacks showed a time course of behaviour of platelet serotonin concentrations consistent with the above interpretation, and at least a temporary rise in plasma water serotonin concentration immediately after the platelet serotonin level began to fall.

Platelet behaviour towards serotonin Several attempts have been made to investigate platelet behaviour towards serotonin during migraine attacks, to try to explain the fall in platelet serotonin concentration at these times. Anthony *et al.*[70] reported that there was no abnormality of serotonin uptake in migraineurs' platelets during and between attacks. However Dalsgaard-Neilsen and Genefke[71] found an increased serotonin content of migraineurs' platelets between migraine attacks, and an increased capacity of the platelets to take up the amine. By way of contrast to both of these studies, in what appear to be three reports of the same investigation Carroll *et al.*[72,73] and Coppen *et al.*[74] measured a decreased V_{max} for serotonin uptake by migraineurs' platelets both during and in the few days following migraine attacks. The K_m for the uptake was unchanged. Malmgren *et al.*[75,76] had also found a decreased serotonin uptake by migraineurs' platelets while Hanington *et al.*[77] recorded a non-statistically significant decrease in platelet serotonin uptake after migraine attacks and decreased serotonin release from platelets within 3 days of a migraine attack. Malmgren *et al.*[78] found no statistically significant difference in the V_{max} or K_m for platelet serotonin uptake between migraineurs and controls. In a recent careful study in untreated migraineurs, Launay *et al.*[79] and Pradalier and Launay[80] showed no difference between controls and migraineurs in the kinetic parameters of platelet serotonin uptake during headache-free intervals. However during attacks in three migraineurs they showed both the K_m and the V_{max} for serotonin uptake were notably reduced. This reduction in Michaelis–Menten parameter values applied only if the uptake was studied in platelets incubated with the migraineurs' own plasma. Platelet serotonin uptake was normal if the migraineurs' platelets were incubated with control plasma to determine platelet serotonin uptake capacity. Thus the work of Launay *et al.*[79] suggested that some factor which interfered with platelet serotonin uptake was present in migraineurs' plasma during migraine attacks. It supported the majority of the investigators, in that it confirmed that platelet capacity to take up serotonin is reduced during migraine attacks.

There had been earlier intimations of the existence of a circulating factor which might play a potential causative role in migraine by altering platelet function. Anthony *et al.*[70], Lance *et al.*[81], Anthony[54] and Anthony and Lance[82] had obtained evidence consistent with the presence in plasma during migraine attacks of a serotonin-releasing factor (shown by these workers to have a molecular weight below 50 000). Dvilansky *et al.*[83] had demonstrated that during, but not between, migraine attacks, migraineurs' plasma caused serotonin release from the platelets of non-migraineurs. Mück-Šeler *et al.*[60] showed that, when platelets from headache-free migraineurs were incubated with platelet-poor plasma from one migraineur collected during an attack, platelet serotonin concentration fell. However, if the platelets tested were taken from non-migraineurs there was no fall in platelet serotonin content after incubation. Thus not only did there appear to be a platelet-active factor in circulating platelet-poor plasma during migraine attacks, but migraineurs' platelets also seemed to react towards a circulating factor in a way that non-migraineur's platelets did not. It is yet to be established whether or not the circulating factor which produces platelet serotonin release in migraine, and the factor which impairs serotonin uptake (referred to in the preceding paragraph), are identical.

Superficial temporal artery serotonin receptors Skärby *et al.*[84] found no difference in the responsiveness of serotonin receptors in migraineurs' temporal arteries, biopsied in the intervals between attacks, and in a normal person's temporal arteries.

3.1.2.2 Central nervous system serotonin

As was indicated in Section 2.3, for over a decade it has been hypothesised that depletion of central nervous system neurotransmitter serotonin may be responsible for migraine. After several weeks administration of *p*-chlorophenylalanine to man, a procedure which might be expected to deplete central nervous system serotonin by inhibiting its synthesis, an experience of diffuse pain over much of the body develops[85]. There has therefore been speculation that a more restricted depletion of the neurotransmitter in the serotoninergic pathway descending from the midbrain raphe to the spinal trigeminal nucleus might produce, or at least augment, head pain in migraine. The cause of such a restricted distribution of the postulated serotonin depletion is as yet unexplained, though there have been suggestions that brain stem ischaemia may be a cause[86]. Welch *et al.*[87] showed that unilateral carotid artery occlusion in gerbils caused decreased serotonin concentrations in both cerebral hemispheres, and increased sensitivity to pain developed. Crook[88] stated that brain serotonin depletion caused increased sensitivity of the vomiting centre. The line of argument attributing serotonin depletion to ischaemia carries the implication that the pain element of migraine is a secondary phenomenon, consequent on primary vascular alterations.

So far as we are aware, there is no direct observational evidence that depleted brain serotonin concentrations are present during human migraine though certain authors have suggested that such changes occur[88]. There is no animal model of migraine, and it seems unlikely that direct evidence of brain stem serotonin concentration changes during migraine attacks in humans could be obtained in the foreseeable future. At the most, what might be obtained would be indirect, and possibly ambiguous, evidence from examination of serotonin precursor and serotonin metabolite levels in CSF. So far, the only information available relevant to this latter possibility is the finding of Hyppä and Kangasnemi[67] that CSF 5-hydroxyindoleacetic acid concentrations showed no statistically significant changes in 18 migraine sufferers studied at several stages of migraine attacks and also when headache-free.

Thus at present we lack evidence that brain serotonin levels are altered in migraine attacks.

3.1.2.3 Alimentary tract and pineal serotonin (and related indoles)

No information is available as to what happens to the major quantity of serotonin in the body, that which is contained in the wall of the alimentary tract. Nor is there information about pineal serotonin or other pineal indoles in migraine. However, Papavasilou *et al.*[89] found that oral melatonin therapy given to patients with Parkinsonism provoked attacks of migraine in four of eleven persons so treated.

3.1.3 Interpretation of the serotonin changes in migraine

A simple interpretation of the combination of (i) the now well established finding of a decreased platelet serotonin content during migraine attacks, (ii) the less adequately proven increase in serotonin metabolite excretion in urine at the same time, and (iii) the alterations in platelet serotonin uptake and release during and around the time of migraine attacks, would be as follows:

(a) an as yet unidentified factor whose source is unknown is taken up by circulating platelets; this uptake causes these platelets to release part of their serotonin content and at the same time may possibly impede further serotonin uptake by platelets;
(b) the released serotonin temporarily raises the plasma water serotonin concentration (a change not yet demonstrated experimentally) and produces vasoconstrictive phenomena which affect, in particular, the cranial circulation;
(c) the released serotonin in plasma water is degraded by virtue of monoamine oxidase activity in vessels walls, and elsewhere. The resulting increased formation of 5-hydroxyindoleacetic acid leads to increased urinary excretion of this metabolite, while plasma water serotonin levels fall again;
(d) the reduced platelet serotonin content together with reduced concentrations of plasma water serotonin (unproven) cause a reduced capacity to maintain vascular tone. Hence vasodilatation develops.

Thus one might explain the initial vasoconstrictive and subsequent vasodilatory phenomena of migraine. Unfortunately, so simple an interpretation is difficult to sustain on closer examination.

If platelet serotonin is released into circulating plasma, why does its vasoconstrictive effect occur dominantly on the vasculature of a limited part of the brain rather than on the vascular system more generally? There are clinical data consistent with a generalised change in vascular reactivity in migraine, and cerebral blood flow studies suggest that the reduced brain perfusion in classical migraine may be reasonably widespread, though more severe in one brain region than in others. Even so, one would have to accept a locally heightened vasoconstrictive tendency to explain the differential reduction in perfusion of one brain area that may occur in classical migraine. An alternative possibility suggested by Behar *et al.*[90] is that there might be asymmetrical release of serotonin from the carotid bodies into the carotid arteries at the start of migraine attacks. Here may not be the place to consider further the factor, or factors, which might determine this postulated locally augmented vascular reactivity. However it is appropriate to raise a second question at this stage, namely is the magnitude of the platelet serotonin release sufficient to explain the cerebral vasoconstrictive phenomena of migraine? Quantities of serotonin of the order of those likely to be released from platelets in migraine, infused into the carotid system of man, failed to produce cerebral vasoconstrictive changes resembling those of migraine[36]. Further Kimball *et al.*[91] failed to induce migraine attacks by giving serotonin intravenously and injected around the superficial temporal artery in patients with a migraine tendency. Moreover, patients with carcinoid tumours, which release considerable amounts of serotonin into the circulation, do not have an increased tendency to migraine[5] though they occasionally fail to consider the possibility that the circulating platelets of normal persons and migraineurs between attacks may be able to take up so much of the administered, or released, serotonin that insufficient remains in plasma water to have a vascular effect, whereas in migraine attacks platelet serotonin uptake is impaired and therefore administered serotonin tends to remain free in plasma water whence it can influence vascular tone. The arguments also do not allow for the possibility that the circulating factor which alters platelet behaviour towards serotonin during migraine attacks may also influence vascular wall serotonin receptor behaviour towards the amine. Therefore one may not be justified in arguing from the effects of serotonin administered intravenously in persons not suffering from migraine to the effects of serotonin released *in vivo* from migraineurs' platelets. That platelet behaviour towards serotonin should be taken into consideration in assessing effects of the amine, is also suggested by the observation that in migraineurs who develop thrombocytopenia, migraine increases at times when the platelet count falls[93].

It may perhaps be accepted that, if there is a regional peculiarity of cerebral arterial reactivity, platelet release of serotonin into the circulation provides a moderately satisfactory explanation for the cerebral vasoconstrictive phenomena of migraine, particularly if an abnormal platelet-active factor is also present in the circulation simultaneously. However, how adequate is the serotonin release hypothesis set down above as an explanation of the scalp vasodilatory phenomena of migraine? In the first place, there is as yet no satisfactory evidence that plasma water serotonin concentration is abnormally low during the headache phase of migraine. Also, there is no direct evidence in man that circulating serotonin depletion causes vasodilatation. And scalp vasodilatation of itself is not necessarily painful, as mentioned earlier (Section 2.1.1.1). Of course, one should bear in mind the *in vitro* experimental observation that serotonin may have a vasodilating rather than vasoconstricting effect on human temporal arteries in a state of heightened vascular tonus[29]. Is it therefore possible that the combination of raised plasma water serotonin levels and the abnormal circulating factor(s) which act on platelet and possibly vessel-wall serotonin receptors may cause initial scalp vasoconstriction in migraine. Continuing exposure of the contracted vessels to high plasma serotonin levels (perhaps in the presence of declining levels of the unknown circulating factor) may lead to subsequent vasodilatation?

In this connection it may be worth noting that serotonin caused decreased flow through scalp arteriovenous shunts in cats[32], yet Heyck[94] suggested there was increased scalp arteriovenous shunting in migraine. Despite this rather contradictory item of evidence, if serotonin can either constrict or dilate cranial vessels, depending on their previous tonus, the serotonin hypothesis of migraine pathogenesis gains in that it is no longer necessary to postulate a fall in plasma water serotonin level to explain scalp vasodilatation in migraine. However, it has been reported that slow intravenous serotonin infusion during the headache phase of 6 attacks of reserpine-induced migraine in 4 subjects relieved the pain of all the attacks[56]. This observation is not consistent with the hypothesis variant discussed immediately above. There does not appear to have been any subsequent report of this effect of infused serotonin in migraine, and Somerville[65], who worked in the same unit as Anthony, denied the existence of this benefit from serotonin infusion. Therefore one is uncertain whether this line of evidence needs to be considered.

Even if the plasma serotonin changes can account for the scalp vasodilatation of migraine, this vasodilatation of itself does not appear to be a sufficient explanation for the pain of migraine, though it may mediate the pulsatile character of the pain. However serotonin, in combination with bradykinin and certain prostaglandins, is known to be capable of initiating impulse formation in pain nerve endings. If scalp vasodilatation followed a period of scalp vasoconstriction and local scalp ischaemia, serotonin might escape into the perivascular zone from capillaries made abnormally permeable by ischaemia. Together with other nocioceptive chemicals this escaped serotonin would then be in position to contribute to the activation of perivascular pain endings. It is also conceivable that the postulated initial serotonin-induced scalp ischaemia might instigate formation of chemicals which may cause active scalp vasodilatation quite irrespective of any effect of serotonin. This possibility is discussed further in subsequent sections (3.5 and 3.6).

There is obvious difficulty in reconciling the occurrence of unilateral headache which is often quite localised with any hypothesis of migraine pathogenesis centered on circulatory chemical alterations. As mentioned earlier, Behar *et al.*[90] proposed an interesting possibility relevant to this point in relation to circulating serotonin and migraine – namely that there could be asymmetrical release of the amine from the carotid bodies into the cranial circulation during migraine. These workers found there was asymmetry in the serotonin contents of the carotid bodies of man. For this hypothesis variant to be taken further it would be desirable to carry out direct measurements of carotid plasma water serotonin content on each side during migraine attacks.

The attractive cerebral nervous system serotonin hypothesis of migraine pathogenesis has already been discussed (Sections 2.3 and 3.1.2.2). Unfortunately the hypothesis is almost totally lacking in any biochemical foundation based on experimental data. However it is interesting to speculate whether the unidentified circulating factor which alters platelet serotonin uptake and release during migraine might also cause release of brain serotonin and thus produce depleted levels of serotonin for neurotransmission. This would link the vascular and central nervous serotonin hypotheses, and would provide a basis for a central amplification of vascular type pain produced peripherally. However, to enter the brain the circulating factor would have to be capable of crossing the blood – brain barrier in the region of the brain stem raphe. Until the chemical nature of the circulating factor is determined there appears little point in taking this line of speculation further. The sort of molecule one might anticipate would be a strong candidate for the role of circulating factor capable of displacing serotonin from platelets would be another amine, possibly an indolealkylamine, but such a molecule would be unlikely to cross the blood – brain barrier easily. Bruyn[95] suggested that it might be a 130 – 140 aminoacid-containing peptide from the hypothalamus, without indicating how he arrived at this possibility.

Willoughby[96] was interested in the question of migraine and penetration of the blood – brain barrier from the reverse direction. He suggested that circulating serotonin might traverse the blood – brain barrier in regions when the barrier is defective, e.g. parts of the hypothalamus, and might act there to produce the vegetative symptoms of migraine.

The role of circulating serotonin in the production of migraine would be more easily assessed if reliable measurement of the time course of plasma water serotonin concentrations before, during and after migraine attacks were carried out, and if measurements of plasma and urine conjugated and unconjugated 5-hydroxyindoleacetic acid were available. Yet, in terms of currently available knowledge, the described serotonin changes in plasma do go some way to providing a biochemical basis for migraine attacks.

3.2 CATECHOLAMINES AND RELATED SUBSTANCES

3.2.1 Biology

3.2.1.1 Formation

The catecholamines are derivatives of the aromatic aminoacids phenylalanine and tyrosine. Analogous series of non-hydroxylated and mono-hydroxylated (i.e. phenolic) amines exist. The relevant biosynthetic pathways for catecholamines and phenolic amines are shown in Figures 3.4 and 3.5.

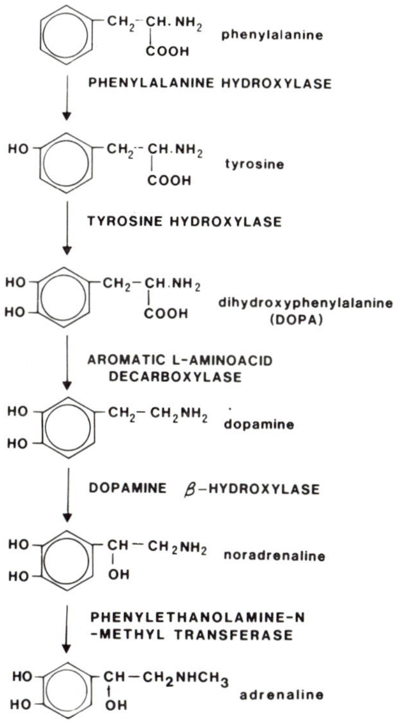

Figure 3.4 Catecholamine biosynthesis

The rate-limiting enzyme in catecholamine formation appears to be tyrosine hydroxylase. Aromatic l-aminoacid decarboxylase appears capable of decarboxylating a number of substrates, including the serotonin precursor 5-hydroxytryptophan, as well as dihydroxyphenylalanine (DOPA) and tyrosine.

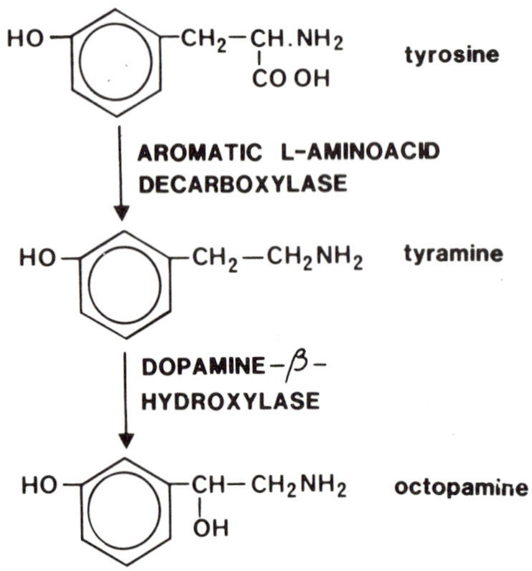

Figure 3.5 Phenolic amine biosynthesis

3.2.1.2 Metabolism

The catecholamines and their lower hydroxylated (phenolic) homologues are metabolised along two pathways, one involving *O*-methylation and the other oxidative deamination. The relevant enzymes are (i) catechol-*O*-methyl transferase, and (ii) monoamine oxidase, respectively. The pathways concerned are illustrated for dopamine and for noradrenaline in Figures 3.6 and 3.7 respectively. Analogous pathways exist for the other aromatic amines mentioned above.

The preferred pathway for noradrenaline metabolism is towards methoxy-hydroxy-phenylglycol in the central nervous system of man[97], and towards vanillylmandelic acid in peripheral tissues. The amines themselves, and their metabolites, are excreted in urine mainly as conjugates, chiefly sulphates formed in a reaction catalysed by the enzyme phenosulphotransferase (Section 4.3.1.3).

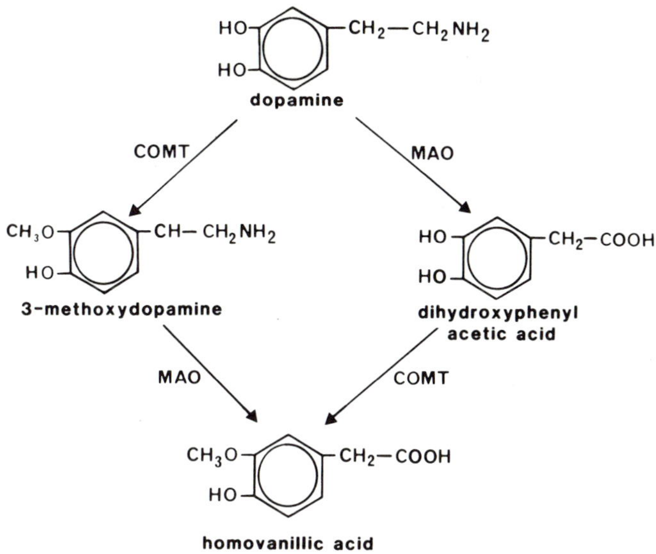

Figure 3.6 Dopamine metabolism

3.2.1.3 Sites of occurrence

The catecholamines and phenolic amines are formed within the central and peripheral nervous systems, and in the adrenal medulla (which embryologically is a development of postganglionic autonomic neurons).

Dopamine is a specific neurotransmitter in certain regions of the central nervous system, notably the nigro-striatal pathway, the hypothalamus, certain areas of the medulla oblongata near the floor of the fourth ventricle and also in projections from the ventral midbrain tegmentum to the limbic cortex and related limbic structures. Dopamine also appears to be a neurotransmitter in the retina. Specific dopamine receptors occur in the renal vascular bed, on sympathetic ganglion cells, in the carotid body, and on presynaptic noradrenergic nerve terminals. Elsewhere in the body dopamine appears to be a metabolic intermediate in noradrenaline formation. There are at least two types of central nervous system dopamine receptor, and possibly more[98]. The matter of subtypes of dopamine receptor is currently under active investigation, but it seems agreed that the D_1 type receptors are adenylate cyclase linked, while the other type (or types) are not. Dopamine does not appear to play a neurotransmitter role in the peripheral nervous system.

In the central nervous system many noradrenergic neurons appear to have their cell bodies in the locus coeruleus in the pons. From this nucleus noradrenergic axons radiate caudally to the cerebellum, brain stem and spinal cord, and rostrally to the cortex, thalamus and hypothalamus. Other noradrenergic neurons occur in the lateral tegmental area, and appear to project in a distribution similar to that of locus coeruleus neurons. In the peripheral nervous system noradrenaline is the neurotransmitter at the terminals of postganglionic sympathetic neurons. There are two main types of noradrenergic receptor, α and β, determined by pharmacological consideration, and two recognised subtypes of each, designated α_1 and α_2, and β_1 and β_2.

Adrenaline is now known to occur in the central nervous system in neurons in the the lateral tegmental area and the dorsal medulla oblongata. Axons from these areas project to the hypothalamus, the dorsal vagal nucleus, locus

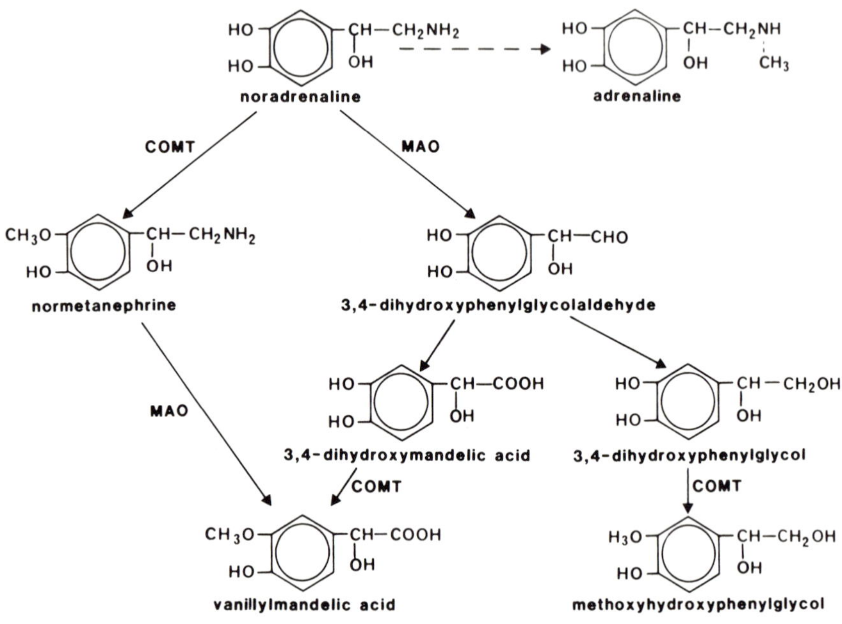

Figure 3.7 Noradrenaline metabolism

coeruleus, intermediolateral column of the spinal cord and the region around the fourth ventricle. The amine is a neurotransmitter in postganglionic sympathetic neurons in some species. It is also formed in the adrenal medulla.

The phenolic amines appear to be present in the central nervous system, but their distributions have been subjected to relatively little study, as yet.

Catecholamines formed in the central nervous system are prevented from entering the blood stream by the blood–brain barrier (which also prevents catecholamines from entering the brain from the circulation). However catecholamines released at peripheral nervous system terminals and catecholamines formed in the adrenal medulla are not excluded from the circulation and attain measurable concentrations there. The circulating catecholamines occur as such, or as conjugates, which in man appear to be entirely sulphates[99]. More than 95% of the dopamine in plasma is present as conjugates[100]. Noradrenaline concentrations in plasma are commonly taken as a measure of contemporaneous peripheral sympathetic activity, and adrenaline concentrations as a measure of adrenal medullary functioning. The origin of circulating dopamine is still uncertain[100], though the adrenal medulla may make a contribution. Normal values for concentrations of the circulating unconjugated catecholamines are:

dopamine: 29 ± 3 ng/l[101]; 54 ± 4 ng/l[100]; 38 ± 11 ng/l[102]
noradrenaline: 200 – 250 ng/l or 304 – 390 ng/l, depending on the type of assay[103]: 292 ± 49 ng/l[101]; 201 ± 50 ng/l[102].
adrenaline: 57 ± 18 ng/l [104]: 81 ± 35 ng/l[101]; 23 ± 4 ng/l[102].

However these concentrations, particularly those of noradrenaline, are very sensitive to the influence of stress, exercise and body position in space[102,103].

The catecholamines also occur in platelets, mainly in the form of sulphate conjugates. The unconjugated catecholamines are present in platelets in concentration ratios similar to those which apply for these substances in plasma water, but at concentrations approximately one thousandth of those of platelet unconjugated serotonin levels[3]. The circulating catecholamines are actively taken up into platelets, which contain little activity of the enzymes necessary for catecholamine synthesis.

Urinary dopamine concentrations are higher than those of noradrenaline, despite plasma dopamine levels being lower than those of noradrenaline. This suggests the possibility that the kidneys may secrete dopamine into the urine.

For convenience, the effects of the various catecholamines are considered separately.

3.2.1.4 Effects of noradrenaline

The l-isomer is more active biologically than its d-counterpart. Noradrenaline is an agonist at α- and β_1-receptors, but has little effect on β_2-type receptors. Noradrenaline given systemically constricts most vascular beds, but increases coronary and adipose tissue blood flow[105]. According to Saxena[33] noradrenaline acts on α-receptors to constrict extracranial and intracranial arterioles and larger arteries, but also has effects in the opposite direction by acting on vascular β-adrenoceptors. However cerebral circulatory autoregulation may offset the consequences of these changes in the intact animal. In man, intracarotid injection of noradrenaline does not alter cerebral blood flow[35].

Noradrenaline causes hyperglycaemia. It promotes platelet aggregation and, given intravenously in experimental animals, causes vomiting[106].

There is some evidence that central nervous system noradrenergic neurotransmission may be involved in the production of sleep, and in the control of mood. The pial blood vessels receive a (constrictor) noradrenergic innervation originating in the locus coeruleus (Section 2.3).

In the peripheral nervous system noradrenergic neurotransmission relaxes alimentary tract smooth muscle (activating both α- and β- receptors), increases myocardial contraction and heart rate (β_1), constricts arterioles in most tissues (α- and β_1-receptors), relaxes urinary bladder muscle (β), promotes glycogenolysis and gluconeogenesis in the liver (α, β_2), causes lipolysis (α, β_1) and promotes melatonin synthesis in the pineal (β-receptors).

3.2.1.5 *Effects of adrenaline*

As with noradrenaline, the l-isomer of adrenaline is more active than the d-isomer. In its activity it tends to be more potent than noradrenaline at α-adrenoceptors, and also at β_2-receptors. Given intravenously it raises blood pressure by increasing myocardial contractility and heart rate, and by constricting many peripheral vascular beds (particularly the arterioles and veins), though coronary and muscle blood flows increase. At doses sufficient to raise blood pressure, cerebral blood flow is also increased by adrenaline administration. However, Olesen and Skinhoj[35] found that intracarotid injection of adrenaline in man did not alter cerebral blood flow. Skin, mucosal and renal blood flows are reduced. Gastrointestinal, bladder and bronchial muscle are relaxed. Hyperglycaemia may occur because of glycolysis and increased gluconeogenesis, with decreased insulin secretion. Free fatty acid levels in the circulation are increased by virtue of stimulation of β_1-type adrenoceptors.

Adrenaline promotes platelet aggregation.

The function of the adrenergic neurons which occur in the central nervous system is as yet uncertain.

3.2.1.6 *Effects of dopamine*

Given intravenously, dopamine acts as an agonist at cardiac β_1- receptors, increasing myocardial contractility. It increases systolic but not diastolic blood pressure, dilating the renal and mesenteric vascular beds but having a mild constrictor effect on other vascular beds. It increases glomerular filtration rate. The amine is thought to act on α-type vascular noradrenaline receptors, though there is suspicion that there may be specific blood vessel dopamine receptors at which the amine has a vasodilator effect[107]. In dogs lower concentrations of intravenously administered dopamine increase cerebral blood flow, but higher concentrations decrease the flow[108].

Dopamine appears to have a weak aggregatory action on platelets, acting via platelet α-adrenoceptors[109].

As a central neurotransmitter, dopamine in the nigrostriatal pathway decreases muscle tone and speeds the initiation of voluntary movement. Its deficiency leads to Parkinsonian rigidity, bradykinesis and loss of physiological associated movements. It seems possible that excessive dopaminic neurotransmission in the limbic system is related to the thought disorder of schizophrenia. Dopaminic neurotransmission in the hypothalamus mediates release of prolactin from the pituitary into the circulation.

3.2.2 Catecholamine changes in migraine

Hsu *et al.*[110,111] reported a rise in mean plasma noradrenaline levels from 0.499 ± 0.040 to 0.664 ± 0.050 μg/l some 3 hours before a group of migrainous subjects awoke with headache already present. More or less contemporaneously Fog-Moller *et al.*[112] reported the seemingly contrary finding of a decline in mean plasma noradrenaline concentration prior to migraine attacks, though with a subsequent increase to levels somewhat above normal during the attacks. Plasma adrenaline concentrations were unchanged throughout these events. Subsequently Anthony[113] confirmed the presence of a rise in plasma noradrenaline concentration during migraine attacks. The levels rose by a mean of 29.9% in a group of ten of his patients, some elevation occurring in all subjects. However, he found that mean plasma adrenaline level fell during the migraine attacks. In earlier studies Curran *et al.*[44] found increased urinary excretion of the noradrenaline metabolite vanillylmandelic acid during migraine attacks, whereas Curzon[50] failed to find any consistent relation between the two. Nattero[52] reported that urinary vanillylmandelic acid excretion was increased during menstrual migraine, though not to a statistically significant extent.

There do not appear to be any published data on plasma dopamine concentrations during migraine. Our own as yet unpublished work on platelet-rich plasma has shown a noticeable and consistent rise in dopamine concentration which begins after migraine has been clinically apparent for an hour or so. Plasma dopamine concentrations had reverted to baseline values by 24 hours from the end of the migraine. Unfortunately we have no data as to the behaviour of plasma dopamine levels prior to the onset of the attacks, and no estimations of dopamine concentrations in platelet-free plasma. Sicuteri *et al.*[114] suggested that central nervous system dopamine receptor hypersensitivity might explain their observation that patients who tended to faint during migraine attacks had blood pressures that were more sensitive to the effects of oral bromocriptine (a central dopamine agonist) than migraineurs who did not faint during attacks; this increased blood pressure sensitivity could be reversed by the administration of dopamine antagonist domperidone. Kangasniemi *et al.*[115] noted a rise in CSF levels of the dopamine metabolite homovanillic acid both during migraine attacks and in the post-headache period.

Many years ago Wolff[116] described the results of an intravenous infusion of noradrenaline in four persons subject to headache. The infusions were continued for up to 3 hours, the infusion rate being sufficient to cause detectable extracranial arterial and conjunctival vessel constriction. No headaches developed during or after the infusions. However, during migraine headache attacks, noradrenaline infusion considerably diminished the severity of the pain or abolished it in 93 of 116 attacks in 35 patients. In general, the more severe the pain the longer the delay before benefit occurred after noradrenaline infusion. The delay ranged in duration from 20 to 160 minutes.

3.2.3 Interpretation of the catecholamine changes in migraine

Hsu *et al.*[110,111] and Fog-Moller *et al.*[112] have produced conflicting evidence as to the behaviour of plasma noradrenaline levels prior to the onset of migraine. It is important that this conflict be reconciled. It has, for instance, been suggested that increased plasma noradrenaline levels in the premonitory phase could promote platelet aggregation, and increased platelet aggregation is known to occur in migraineurs, at least in clinical attacks (Section 2.2). This increased platelet aggregation could cause the aggregating platelets to release serotonin, promoting further platelet aggregation and setting in train the serotonin changes discussed in Section 3.1 which appear to contribute to the phenomena of migraine. However this whole line of reasoning becomes quite untenable if the finding of Hsu *et al.*[111] is not confirmed. Further, this line of argument ignores the failure of Wolff[116] to induce migraine in susceptible persons by infusing noradrenaline.

The rise in plasma noradrenaline level during attacks seems more securely documented, though it is uncertain whether this represents a contributing element to the vascular changes of migraine, or is simply a consequence of sympathetic overactivity related to the stress experienced by the migraineur during his attacks. Anthony[55,113] appeared to favour the latter interpretation. However, he made the point that altered sympathetic activity and raised noradrenaline levels could cause other biochemical changes relevant to migraine, as will be discussed later (Section 4.2).

The raised plasma noradrenaline levels that are reported during the headache phase of migraine seem unlikely to contribute directly towards the extracranial vasodilatation present at this stage of the disorder, in view of the known vasoconstrictor actions of the amine. Conceivably these raised noradrenaline levels might help perpetuate the tendency to increased platelet aggregation during attacks, and so help maintain serotonin release into plasma water during attacks. Alternatively, bearing in mind Wolff's[116] description of how noradrenaline infusions relieved migraine, the reported elevation of plasma noradrenaline levels during migraine headaches could perhaps be seen as a homeostatic mechanism favouring the termination of attacks. At the same time the delays that Wolff reported between the commencement of noradrenaline infusions and the appearance of pain relief suggest that direct noradrenaline-mediated vasoconstriction may not have been responsible for the relief of pain. Rather some less directly-acting and more delayed mechanism may have been involved.

When there is conflict between the findings of Fog-Muller *et al.*[112] and Anthony[113] as to the behaviour of plasma adrenaline levels during migraine, one has no secure basis on which to assign a role in migraine to this catecholamine.

The timing of the plasma dopamine changes in migraine that we have described above suggests that they are secondary. If they are paralleled by an increase in dopamine concentrations in plasma water it is conceivable that this could contribute to the production of nausea and vomiting in migraine. Although dopamine is too polar a molecule to cross the blood – brain barrier, the barrier is defective over the area postrema in the floor of the fourth ventricle (the 'vomiting centre'), and here dopamine is a neurotransmitter. During levodopa therapy for parkinsonism, prior to the use of the aminoacid combined with peripherally acting inhibitors of aromatic L-aminoacid decarboxylase, vomiting following intake of the drug was common, and at this stage plasma dopamine levels would be expected to be high. However, we would prefer not to take the interpretation of our plasma dopamine findings in migraine too far until we also measure the amine in plasma water. It seems to us that the suggestion of Sicuteri *et al.*[114] that central dopamine receptors are hypersensitive in certain migraineurs needs to be corroborated by other lines of evidence before it is considered further.

It is perhaps a pity that more measurements have not been made on urinary (and plasma) vanillylmandelic acid and homovanillic acid in migraine. Such data could help interpret the mechanism of the altered plasma noradrenaline and dopamine concentrations in the disorder. It could also be informative to see if methoxyhydroxyphenylglycol excretion alters; if this occurred it could raise the possibility that central nervous system catecholamine metabolism is changed. It might also be important to examine the detailed time course of alterations in amine concentrations in both plasma water and in platelets during attacks; if platelets during migraine have an impaired capacity for taking up and retaining serotonin, they may also behave differently towards catecholamines at this time.

While circulating catecholamine changes do appear to develop during migraine attacks, they are not yet as firmly documented as they might be. The interpretation of the catecholamine changes is of necessity somewhat tentative. However on the whole it appears unlikely on the basis of presently available evidence that these changes play a major causative role in initiating migraine attacks. They may be, at least in part, a consequence of migraine attacks, though they could contribute towards the production of some of the secondary phenomena in the disorder.

3.3 ENZYMES INVOLVED IN INDOLEALKYLAMINE AND CATECHOLAMINE METABOLISM

Two enzymes involved in serotonin and catecholamine metabolism have been studied in migraine. These enzymes are (i) monoamine oxidase, which has been investigated at some length, and (ii) dopamine-β-hydroxylase. It will be more convenient to discuss these enzymes separately. Monoamine oxidase is extensively involved in indolealkylamine and catecholamine metabolism, while dopamine-β-hydroxylase appears to have the specific function of catalysing the conversion of dopamine to noradrenaline.

3.3.1 Monoamine oxidase

3.3.1.1 Biology

Function Monoamine oxidase (MAO; EC 1.4.3.4) is a mitochondrial enzyme which catalyses the oxidative deamination of a variety of aromatic or aliphatic primary amines. The general reaction catalysed is:

$$R\text{-}CH_2.NH_2 \xrightarrow{MAO} R\text{-}\overset{\overset{O}{\parallel}}{C}H + NH_3$$

The aldehyde product of the reaction then undergoes oxidation to a carboxylic acid, or reduction to a glycol. These latter reactions appear to be very rapid, so that the existence of the aldehyde intermediate is transient.

Substrate specificity Two types of monoamine oxidase are commonly designated, as determined by the relative specificity of the enzyme towards certain amine substrates and by the selectively of its inhibition. This subdivision into functional types of enzyme may be more appropriate for the enzyme in certain accessible tissues, e.g. circulating platelets, than for the enzyme in less accessible organs such as the brain, and in the *in vivo* situation[117]. However, it is in one such accessible tissue, namely platelets, that monoamine oxidase has been studied in relation to migraine.

The types of monoamine oxidase, with their substrate and inhibitor specificities in man, are shown in Table 3.1.

Table 3.1

	Monoamine oxidase	
Substrates	*Type A*	*Type B*
5-Hydroxytryptamine	+	-
Tryptamine		+
Tyramine	+	+
Phenylethylamine	-	+
Dopamine	+	+
Noradrenaline	+	-
Benzylamine	-	+
Methylhistamine	-	+
Kynuramine	+	+
Methyl histamine	-	+
Inhibitors		
Clorgyline	+	-
Amphetamine	+(r)	
Harmaline	+(r)	
Mixelitine	+(r)	
Deprenyl	-	+
Imipramine	-	+(r)
Amitriptyline	-	+(r)

(r) = reversible
(information is not readily available for those items left blank).

Monoamine oxidase distribution Monoamine oxidase is widely distributed in the body, occurring in certain brain regions (particularly those involved in catecholaminergic and serotoninergic neurotransmission), in the liver, the intestinal wall (type 'A' only[118]), in blood vessel walls and, within the blood stream, in circulating platelets and leukocytes (type B in both[119]) and in granulocytes (type A). Another deaminating enzyme, benzylamine oxidase, is present in plasma and in blood vessel walls, but is absent from platelets[120].

Platelet monoamine oxidase Platelet monoamine oxidase is a mitochondrial enzyme[3]. It is an electrophoretically homogeneous protein with a molecular weight of 23 500[121] and is of functional type 'B' only[122]. Thus it does not catalyse the degradation of noradrenaline or serotonin. Its activity tends to undergo a degree of diurnal variation[123]. Platelet monoamine oxidase activity is said to vary with the phase of the menstrual cycle, the activity being maximal at the time of ovulation[124], though this has been denied[125], to be higher in women than men[126], and to be increased in cases of unipolar depression[125]. Monoamine oxidase activity levels were reported to be greater in freshly released platelets[127] and in larger platelets[120,125], though Peatfield *et al.*[128] failed to confirm this finding. There is no correlation between platelet monoamine oxidase activity and platelet serotonin release in response to ADP[129]. Peatfield *et al.*[130] have adduced some preliminary evidence suggesting that platelet monoamine oxidase activity may reflect to some extent whole body activity of the enzyme.

3.3.1.2 Platelet monoamine oxidase changes in migraine

The platelets are the only body component in which monoamine oxidase activity has been studied in relation to migraine. There are now a number of reports that platelet monoamine oxidase activity is reduced during migraine attacks[118,123,131,132,133,134]. As more data have accumulated it has become clear that the fall in platelet monoamine oxidase occurs in males but not in females, and in males it occurs in those with classical rather than common migraine[125,135]. Glover *et al.*[136] had earlier noted that platelet monoamine oxidase activity also tended to be reduced in migraineurs in the interval between attacks, though the reduction was not statistically significant. They found that platelet monoamine oxidase activity decreased further during actual migraine attacks. Subsequently Glover *et al.*[135] showed that those migraineurs who had reduced platelet monoamine oxidase levels when first studied also had reduced levels when restudied 4 years later. By way of contrast Thomas[137] failed to find any differences in platelet monoamine oxidase activity between migraineurs in attack-free intervals and control subjects. Nor did Littlewood *et al.*[138], apparently contrary to earlier results from the same group of workers.

Since platelet aggregation increases during migraine attacks, it has been suggested that larger platelets may be selectively segregated from the general circulation. These larger platelets have higher monoamine oxidase contents, according to Sandler *et al.*[125]. Therefore the fall in platelet monoamine oxidase activity during migraine attacks may be due to a preferential retention in the circulation of smaller platelets with lower monoamine oxidase contents rather than due to a change in enzyme content of individual platelets. However, Peatfield *et al.*[128] have shown that (i) platelet monoamine oxidase activity does not correlate with platelet volume, and (ii) platelet size does not differ between migraineurs and control subjects.

Benzylamine oxidase Circulating levels of this enzyme are unchanged in migraine.

3.3.1.3 Interpretation of the platelet monoamine oxidase changes in migraine

The platelet monoamine oxidase changes in migraine appear restricted to one type of the disorder, the 'classical' variety, and within this variety to one sex only. Platelet monoamine oxidase does not catalyse the deamination of the two biogenic amines, serotonin and noradrenaline, which appear most likely to be involved in the pathogenesis of migraine. Therefore one may well ask whether the reported monoamine oxidase changes have relevance to the mechanisms of migraine. In fact as long ago as 1977 Sandler suggested that the monoamine oxidase changes reported in migraine may simply reflect platelet injury, possibly related to the increased platelet aggregation which occurs in migraine attacks. On the whole the monoamine oxidase changes, which when first reported appeared highly pertinent to the question of altered circulating amine activity in migraine, have begun to seem increasingly irrelevant since the substrate specificity of platelet monoamine oxidase has been more widely appreciated, and it has become apparent that the changes are not invariable phenomena in migraineurs.

It is attractive to speculate that the platelet monoamine oxidase changes might parallel monoamine oxidase changes (not necessarily of type B only) in other organs during migraine. If this occurred, impaired gut wall monoamine oxidase activity prior to and during migraine attacks could allow dietary amines which are normally degraded during passage through the intestinal mucosa to reach the circulation intact. There they might competitively displace serotonin from platelets, thus initiating what seem in terms of current knowledge to be the central events of the migraine mechanism. In this way dietary migraine could be explained. However, there is no evidence whatsoever that gut wall monoamine oxidase activity is altered during migraine: the suggestion advanced above is purely speculative.

3.3.2 Dopamine-β-hydroxylase

The enzyme dopamine-β-hydroxylase is a copper-containing protein which occurs in the adrenal medulla, sympathetic nervous system and brain. It appears to be located in the membranes of amine storage granules in axon terminals of the sympathetic nervous system[139]. The enzyme catalyses the oxidation of the β-carbon atom on the alkyl side chain of dopamine, thus forming noradrenaline (Figure 3.4), and structurally related phenolic amines. Dopamine-β-hydroxylase requires molecular oxygen for its action and utilises ascorbic acid as a co-factor.

During sympathetic nervous system activity, as amine storage granules with their noradrenaline contents are released into synaptic clefts, some dopamine-β-hydroxylase is also released and enters the circulation[139]. Serum (or plasma) dopamine-β-hydroxylase activity has come to be regarded as a moderately satisfactory index of contemporaneous sympathetic nervous system activity[140,141]. The enzyme in the circulation does not appear to arise from the adrenals.

Gotoh *et al.*[142] found higher mean serum dopamine-β-hydroxylase activity in a group of 17 migraineurs in the interval between their headache attacks, as compared with 16 subjects with contraction headache and 40 normal 'control' subjects. During attacks of migraine Anthony[113] noted increased serum dopamine-β-hydroxylase activity (mean increase 42%) in all 10 patients he studied. The activity continued to be increased after the headaches ended in his migraineurs.

These findings suggest increased sympathetic nervous system activity in and around the time of migraine attacks. They are in keeping with the belief that raised plasma noradrenaline concentrations during migraine (Section 3.2) reflect heightened sympathetic activity. Thus the two findings are mutually supportive.

3.4 HISTAMINE

3.4.1 Biology

The biology of histamine, from a clinical viewpoint, is described by Beaven[143].

3.4.1.1 Formation

Histamine is formed within the body by decarboxylation of the aminoacid histidine. The enzyme responsible for catalysis of this reaction, histidine decarboxylase, appears to be a substrate specific one, and is not identical with the enzyme that decarboxylates dihydroxyphenylalanine or 5-hydroxytryptophan. Histidine decarboxylase requires pyridoxal phosphate as co-factor.

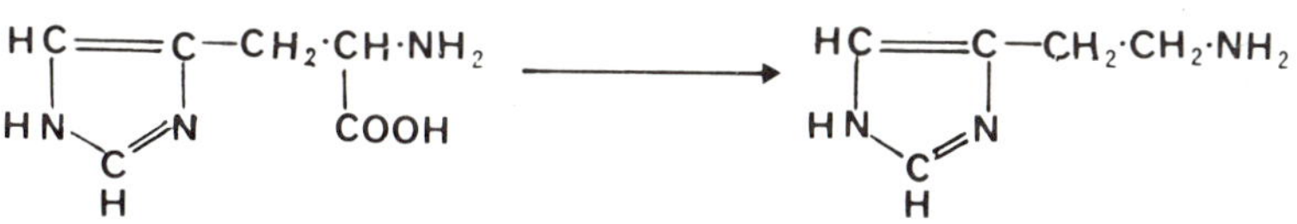

histidine histamine

3.4.1.2 Metabolism

The metabolic degradation of histamine follows two possible routes. Firstly, the amine may be oxidatively deaminated in a reaction catalysed by the enzyme diamine oxidase, and the resulting aldehyde may then be oxidised to imidazole acetic acid, a series of reactions analogous to those undergone by catecholamines and serotonin (though monoamine oxidase is not involved in the case of histamine). Alternatively, histamine may undergo certain conjugation reactions. It is either acetylated at the terminal primary amine group of the alkyl side-chain, or methylated at the secondary amine group in the imidazole ring to form methylhistamine which may itself undergo an oxidative deamination catalysed by monoamine oxidase. The relevant reactions are shown in Figure 3.8.

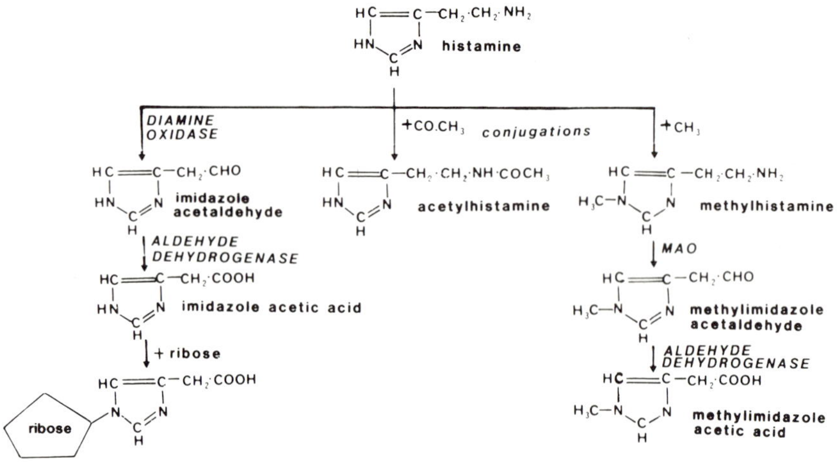

Figure 3.8 Histamine metabolism

Most tissues appear able to degrade histamine, and the overall capacity for the degradation is considerable. Intravenously administered histamine disappears from plasma within a few minutes[143]. Only 1 or 2% of a parenteral histamine dose is excreted unchanged in urine.

3.4.1.3 Sites of occurrence

Histamine occurs in storage granules in mast cells, together with heparin, and in basophil leukocytes. Mast cells occur mostly in perivascular connective tissue. Apart from mast cells, in some species histamine occurs in certain cells in the gastric and intestinal mucosae. In the brain some histamine is present in mast cells[144], but some occurs in nerve terminals of hypothalamic neurons. There is increasing evidence that histamine plays a role as a neurotransmitter in the hypothalamus[145].

Histamine occurs in normal human plasma at a concentration of around 80 μg/l[143], or 2.42 $\pm$ SE 0.17 nmol/l[146] and in platelets at a level of around 1.40 nmol/mg platelet protein[3].

3.4.1.4 Effects

A number of factors (e.g. trauma, burns, infection, immediate hypersensitivity reactions) cause mast cells to release histamine.

Histamine appears to activate two different types of receptor, designated H_1 and H_2 and differentiated by virtue of their sites of occurrence, consequences of activation and responses to agonists and antagonists. Activation of H_1 receptors causes bronchial and alimentary tract contraction. Activation of H_2 receptors enhances gastric acid secretion. H_1 and H_2 receptor activation dilates small blood vessels in the carotid tree[33], an effect mediated via cyclic AMP[147]. Activation of at least H_1 receptors leads to increased permeability of the microcirculation, while activation of H_2 receptors increases the rate and force of cardiac contraction. Histamine also causes pain and itch.

The effects of histamine as a central neurotransmitter are not yet adequately explored. Histamine dilates arterio-venous anastomoses[148]. It is a non-competitive inhibitor of platelet serotonin uptake[149].

Wolff, in seeking candidate substances for a role in the pathogenesis of migraine, carried out extensive investigations on the actions of histamine in man. This work was described in detail in the 1963 edition of his monograph[116]. Wolff concluded that, though injection of histamine produced a vascular type of head pain, this was not really migraine. He considered that the histamine-induced pain arose from distension of intracranial vessels, though scalp arteries contributed to the pain to a relatively minor extent. Pickering[150] had reached an essentially similar conclusion. It is unnecessary to examine in detail all the experiments Wolff conducted in this area. Krabbe and Olesen[151] have recently shown that intravenous infusion of histamine does not alter mean cerebral blood flow, measured with ^{133}Xe. From this finding these authors have argued that histamine headache must arise extracranially. However it should be noted that Krabbe and Olesen's[151] experimental procedure did not produce headache in the subjects they studied, unlike the situation in the subjects Wolff[116] investigated. Further, the capacity of the ^{133}Xe method to measure meningeal blood flow is unclear.

3.4.2 Histamine alterations in migraine

As a substance known to be capable of causing vasodilatation, and of producing pain, histamine at first appeared a possible candidate for a role in the biochemical production of migraine. However, Wolff's[116] studies made it a rather inadequate candidate.

There are some experimental data bearing on histamine changes which have been reported in human migraine. Sicuteri[152] noted mast cell degranulation during migraine, and speculated that this could lead to histamine release into the circulation. Thonnard-Neumann[153] found increased numbers of basophil leukocytes and more degranulated basophils in blood taken from the temple and ear lobe on the side affected by headache during migraine attacks, when compared with blood taken from the opposite ear lobe. This suggested increased histamine (and possibly heparin) release on the affected side during migraine. Sjaastad and Sjaastad[154] noted an increased amount of histamine in 24 hour urine collections in 5 out of a group of 11 migraine sufferers in the intervals between headache attacks. Of itself, this finding is difficult to interpret in the absence of data about simultaneous plasma histamine levels, and the urinary excretions of histamine metabolites. In contrast, Loisy *et al.*[155] found normal urinary excretion of histamine in migraineurs in the interval between attacks, but increased excretion of the histamine metabolite methyl-imidazole acetic acid. Anthony and Lance[156] in an investigation of a group of ten subjects noted increased plasma histamine levels during attacks of migraine in six, unaltered levels in one, and decreased levels in three. The mean levels tended to be higher in the 24 hours after attacks than during or before attacks. Zimmerman *et al.*[157] reported the occurrence of increased spontaneous histamine release from leukocytes from migraineurs in the intervals between migraine attacks. In the following year Sanders *et al.*[158] obtained a similar result in non-allergic migraineurs during attacks. It is difficult to know whether the amount of histamine released in such a reaction could explain the reports of increased urinary excretion of histamine or its metabolite, or the post-migraine rise in plasma histamine concentration found by Anthony and Lance[156].

Sicuteri[159] stated that 80% of persons with migraine given a histamine infusion developed an attack within 2 days of the time when the attack was expected, and that histamine given during an attack increased the severity of the pain. He considered that histamine unmasked migraine. However ranitidine, a H_2 histamine-receptor blocking agent, failed as a migraine preventive[160].

Selmaj[161] found that serum from migraineurs caused increased histamine release from blood donor leukocytes.

3.4.3 Interpretation of the histamine changes in migraine

The investigations of Wolff[116] made it seem unlikely that histamine played any causative role in migraine. Subsequent studies of plasma histamine concentrations and histamine metabolism in migraine seem to have been somewhat perfunctory and no clear or consistent pattern of change has emerged from the findings so far reported. The fact that no consistent change in plasma histamine levels appears to occur during migraine attacks is in keeping with Wolff's view that histamine is not causally related to the mechanisms of migraine. If histamine metabolism is altered in migraine, the alteration is probably a consequence of having migraine. Until new evidence appears, it does not appear worth considering further the role of histamine in migraine.

3.5 BRADYKININ AND RELATED OLIGOPEPTIDES

3.5.1 Biology

Several extensive recent reviews of bradykinin and related kinins are available[162,163,164]. The history of studies of the role of kinins in migraine has been described by Goodell[165].

3.5.1.1 Chemistry and formation

Bradykinin is a basic serine oligopeptide (MW 1060) comprising nine aminoacid residues in the sequence shown in Figure 3.9

The closely related oligopeptide kallidin (lysine – bradykinin) has a lysine residue attached by a peptide bond to the arginine residue at the N-terminal of bradykinin. Other kinins, e.g. the so-called neurokinin, exist.

Kinin formation is the culmination of a sequence of biochemical events occurring in blood and other biological fluids. A peptide prekallikrein (MW 130 000) is synthesised in the liver and other viscera and released into the circulation. Here factor XII (Hageman factor), if activated, e.g. by contact with collagen fibrils, reacts with the prekallikrein to form the peptide kallikrein

arginine
proline
proline
glycine
phenylalanine
serine
proline
phenylalanine
arginine-OH

Figure 3.9 Aminoacid residues of bradykinin

(MW 95 000 – 100 000). The Hageman factor activation also activates certain proteases involved in blood clotting, fibrinolysis and reactions involving complement. Kallikrein has the electrophoretic mobility of a γ-globulin, and functions as a proteolytic and esterolytic enzyme. Kallikrein acts on kininogens, a family of plasma α-globulins of molecular weights in the ranges 48 000 – 70 000, and 100 000 – 200 000, to cleave off various kinins, including bradykinin. Thus the sequence of events in Figure 3.10 occurs:

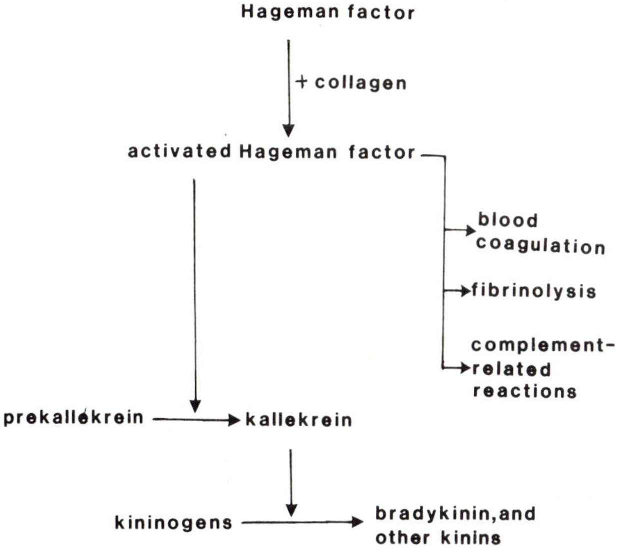

Figure 3.10 Events leading to bradykinin formation

3.5.1.2 Metabolism

The kinins are rapidly inactivated in the circulation and in the lungs. In plasma a carboxypeptidase (kininase I) cleaves the N-terminal arginine residue from the bradykinin oligopeptide, and in the lungs another carboxypeptidase (kininase II) cleaves the bond between the proline and phenylalanine residues at the N-terminal of the molecule (Figure 3.11).

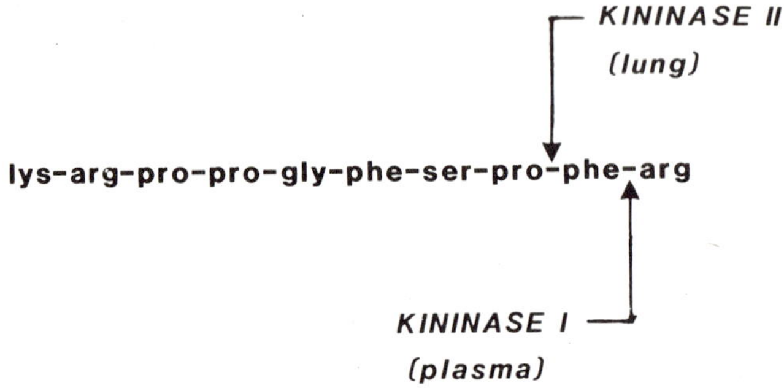

Figure 3.11 Sites of enzymatic inactivation of bradykinin

These enzymatic processes inactivate the kinins very efficiently, the half-life of intravenously administered bradykinin in man being estimated at 0.3 – 0.4 min. Lysine – bradykinin is somewhat more resistant to the peptidases than is bradykinin.

Kallikreins are inactivated much more slowly than kinins.

3.5.1.3 Occurrence

Effectively, the kinins are local hormones because of their highly efficient inactivation in the lungs, and in plasma. They tend to be present mainly at or near their sites of formation. The distribution of bradykinin is restricted to the blood-stream since the oligopeptide is too polar a molecule to achieve easy transit out of the circulation.

Now that reasonably satisfactory radioimmunoassays are available, it appears that plasma bradykinin levels in the normal are below 3 μg/l.[162], and in the range 0.40 – 0.46 μg/l[166].

Kallikreins occur in the pancreas, kidney, intestine, salivary and sweat glands.

3.5.1.4 Effects

Bradykinin and the other kinins so far studied seem to have generally similar effects. Bradykinin and its relatives appear to act on at least two types of receptors (B_1 and B_2). Bradykinin seems to act more potently on B_2 receptors and lysine – bradykinin on B_1 receptors. Additionally, the kinins appear to facilitate prostaglandin formation, in particular prostacyclin (PGI_2) formation[167]. This latter finding makes it necessary to consider to what extent the kinins act directly, and to what extent via the agency of prostaglandins.

Bradykinin is a potent vasodilator (? due to an effect of prostaglandins[168]). It dilates various human cranial arteries[169], though it can constrict arteries in other animal species. In dogs it dilates the external carotid system[22]. It lowers blood pressure, decreases vascular resistance and increases vascular permeability[170]. Urine excretion of conjugated 5-hydroxyindoleacetic acid is increased after a bradykinin infusion[38]. Kallikreins and kinins can produce many of the manifestations of inflammation, and local kinin production is increased in areas of experimentally produced inflammation. Kallikreins are present in leukocytes.

The kinins produce pain if applied near pain nerve endings, or administered intra-arterially[170] but not if given intravenously[171] due to their rapid inactivation in plasma and the lungs. This pain-producing effect of bradykinin is potentiated by serotonin.

The syndrome of hyperbradykininism in man presents with orthostatic hypotension, facial erythema, ecchymoses and purplish discoloration of the legs[172].

3.5.2 Kinin changes in migraine

There are suggestions that bradykinin may be involved in the pathogenesis of migraine[173] though we cannot trace any record of direct measurements of plasma bradykinin levels in the disorder. Sicuteri[152] stated that mast cells degranulated during migraine, releasing kinin – forming enzymes into the bloodstream. Greppi and Sicuteri[174] found reduced plasma kininogen levels during the latter stages of migraine attacks, a change consistent with increased formation of bradykinin and other kinins. Chapman and Wolff[175] noted raised CSF bradykinin levels during migraine in only two of 19 subjects. Kangasniemi *et al.*[51] found evidence of increased bradykinin amidase activity in CSF during and after migraine attacks. Later, these same workers reported evidence of breakdown of bradykinin in the CSF of 12 of 46 migraine sufferers, but in only 2 of 10 control subjects[176]. Bradykinin is a powerful arterial dilator (an action possibly mediated via prostacyclin), possesses pain producing potential and can increase vascular permeability. Therefore bradykinin would seem a promising candidate for a role in the migraine mechanism, if one accepts the vascular hypothesis of migraine pathogenesis. Because bradykinin is so efficiently inactivated on passage through the lungs, it would probably be necessary to measure bradykinin in jugular venous blood taken from the side of migraine headache to try to ascertain if bradykinin played a role in the disorder.

It should perhaps be noted that migraine does not seem to be a conspicuous feature of the syndrome of hyperbradykininism in man. This syndrome appears to present with hypotensive manifestations. However, it may be that the situation in this syndrome is not really comparable with that in migraine. In hyperbradykininism the lungs (with their bradykinin-inactivating capacity) are interposed between the sites of bradykinin production and the cranial circulation where any action that bradykinin had in migraine might be expected to occur. Sicuteri *et al.*[170] reported that intracarotid injection of bradykinin caused ipsilateral head pain. Lower bradykinin doses were required to produce this effect when migraine was present than in the headache-free interval. With intracarotid administration one might anticipate that bradykinin would reach the cranial circulation before it was inactivated. Elkind *et al.*[177] mentioned that bradykinin injected around scalp arteries in migraineurs in the headache-free period did not provoke migraine attacks. Friedman[178] also stated that local intradermal injection of bradykinin near the superficial temporal artery did not cause head pain of the vascular type, though it did increase local blood flow.

Wolff and his colleagues[179,180], aware that blister fluid had pain-producing properties, injected such fluid around superficial temporal arteries that had been (painlessly) dilated in response to heating of the subjects' bodies. The blister fluid was first let stand in contact with a glass surface for long enough for bradykinin (and other kinin) formation to occur. In all subjects headache identical with migraine occurred 20 – 60 minutes later, on the side of the injection, but not on the opposite side (which had received a control injection of saline). Following this finding, these workers injected isotonic saline into the area of pain in two subjects during spontaneous migraine attacks. They then aspirated a small volume of fluid from this area and showed that the aspirate had algesic and vasodilating properties. Subsequent studies[116] on subsurface scalp fluid collected by aspiration during migraine attacks were carried out and a bioassay was used to try to identify the vasoactive, algesic principle. Wolff and his co-workers were able to determine that a substance with many of the properties of bradykinin or plasma kinin was present in the scalp fluid. However, it was concluded that the substance was not identical with plasma kinin. It was considered to be an allied peptide kinin, and named 'neurokinin'. Its exact nature was not determined chemically. It proved to be a powerful vasodilator which increased capillary permeability and induced pain when injected.

3.5.3 Interpretation of kinin changes in migraine

Wolff's[116] finding of a vasoactive, algesic substance present at the site of head pain during attacks of migraine seems a most important observation. The experimental design employed in Wolff's studies appears impeccable, in terms of the knowledge of two decades ago, and it appears surprising, and regrettable, that the studies have not been repeated to permit the nature of the active substance to be identified by contemporary analytical chemical methods.

In the absence of more exact knowledge of the nature of the vasoactive algesic substance that Wolff found, it may be unwise to attempt to construct any line of argument relating the kinins to migraine. Nevertheless, Wolff's observations should be kept in mind. They may prove critically important in understanding the biochemical pathogenesis of migraine. Undoubtedly bradykinin and its relatives have properties which would allow them to fit very well into the vascular type hypothesis of the migraine mechanism. Further, the involvement of bradykinin (or, by virtue of bradykinin's effect on prostaglandin formation, prostacyclin) would open the possibility that the vasodilation of scalp arteries in migraine was an active process, and not merely a passive effect of loss of serotonin-mediated vasoconstriction.

Even though the changes were not consistently present, Chapman and Wolff's[175] observation of increased protease activity in CSF during migraine, as it were setting the stage for possible biologically active peptide formation, could indicate that kinin formation also occurs around the larger intracranial vessels, where it might play a role in migraine production. Again, this matter needs to be re-evaluated by modern chemical methods.

3.6 PROSTAGLANDINS (EICOSANOIDS)

As yet there is no firm evidence of involvement of prostaglandins in migraine. Knowledge of prostaglandin biology has expanded so recently and so rapidly that there may not have been time for the possible role of prostaglandins in migraine to be explored even reasonably adequately. The properties of the prostaglandins, at least in so far as they affect the vascular system, are such that these substances warrant consideration in any attempted interpretation of the biochemical mechanisms of migraine.

3.6.1 Biology

Numerous accounts of prostaglandin biology exist, in particular relating to the vascular effects of these substances[181]. Because the relevant literature is so voluminous, and the role of prostaglandins in migraine as yet tentative, we have elected to concentrate on the vascular and pain producing effects of these substances in the present account.

3.6.1.1 Formation

The term 'eicosanoid' embraces the prostaglandins themselves, the thromboxanes, the leukotrienes and certain other unsaturated fatty acid derivatives containing a chain of 20 carbon atoms. In popular usage at least the thromboxanes, and sometimes the leukotrienes, are often embraced in the term 'prostaglandins', but we will here follow the more precise terminology.

The eicosanoids are derivatives of the unsaturated essential fatty acid arachidonic acid (all *cis*-5, 8, 11, 14-eicosatetraenoic acid),

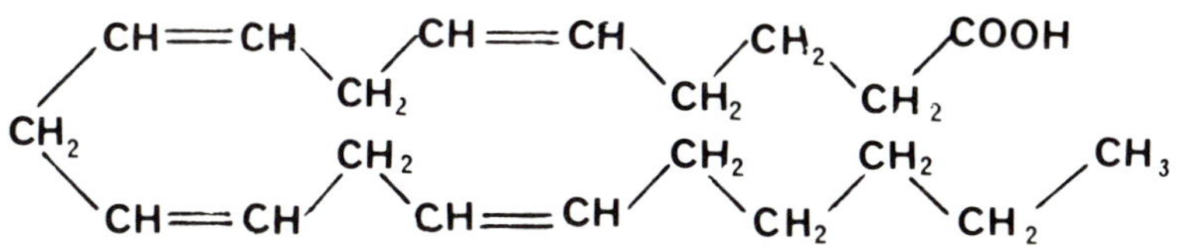

Figure 3.12 Arachidonic acid

the formula for which is often drawn for simplicity (here with numbered C atoms) as follows (Figure 3.13).

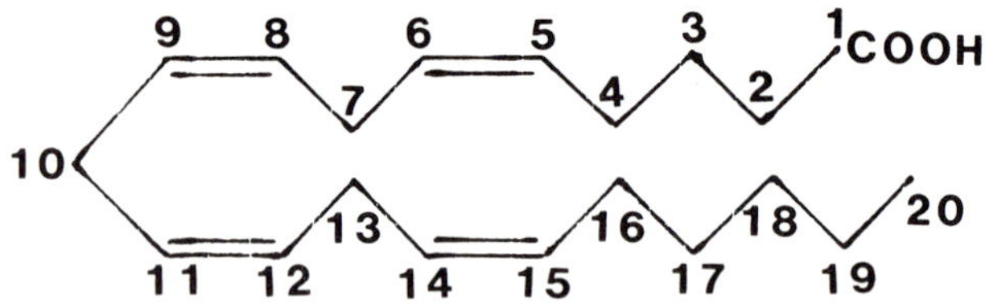

Figure 3.13 Arachidonic acid

Arachidonic acid for eicosanoid formation is provided from cleavage of cell membrane phospholipids, a reaction catalysed by the enzyme phospholipase A_2. This reaction is thought to be the rate-limiting step in eicosanoid production. Phospholipids are phosphorus-containing lipids. Except for sphingomyelins (derivatives of sphingosine) the phospholipids are all glycerol derivatives with the general formula:

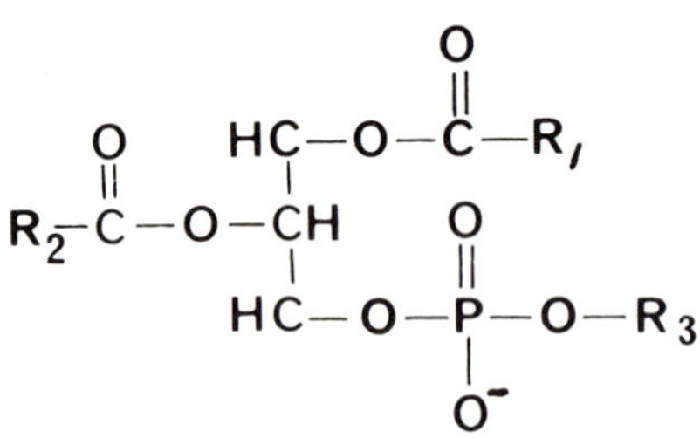

glycerophospholipid

where R_1 and R_2 represent various fatty acids, including arachidonic acid, and R_3 represents ethanolamine, choline, serine or inositol. In sphingomyelins fatty acids are linked through an amide bond to sphingosine, which itself is linked via phosphoric acid to choline. In cell membranes a series of biochemical events occurs (summarised by Wolfe[181]). Factors such as activation of β-adrenergic receptors, contact with immunoglobulins, IgE antigens, mitogens or peptides set the reactions in train and cause phospholipase A_2 to release arachidonic acid, particularly from phosphatidylethanolamine. In platelets other activating factors (e.g. collagen, thrombin, trypsin) cause Ca^{2+}-dependant specific phospholipase C to release arachidonic acid from phosphatidylinositol, through the initial formation of a diacylglycerol:

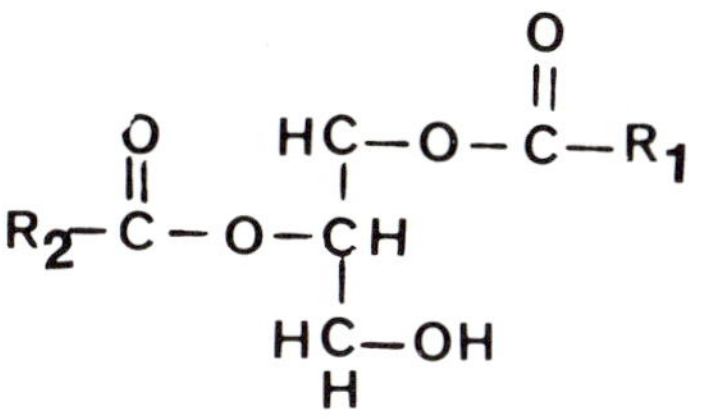

diacylglycerol

The arachidonic acid moiety is subsequently released from this molecule by the hydrolytic action of a lipase. Alternatively the diacylglycerol may be converted to a phosphoric ester (phosphatidic acid) on which phospholipase A_2 may subsequently act to release arachidonic acid.

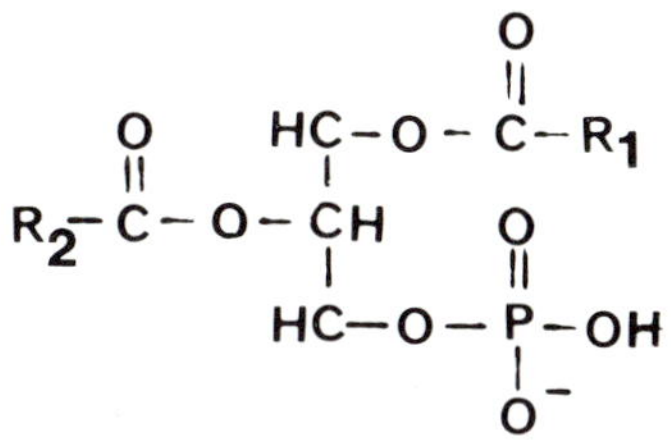

phosphatidic acid

A similar reaction is believed to occur in neutrophil leukocytes.

The released arachidonic acid may then follow a number of reaction pathways which appear to be differentially developed in different types of cells. The general pattern of the pathways is shown in outline in Figure 3.14, and individual pathways are then considered in more detail, where relevant.

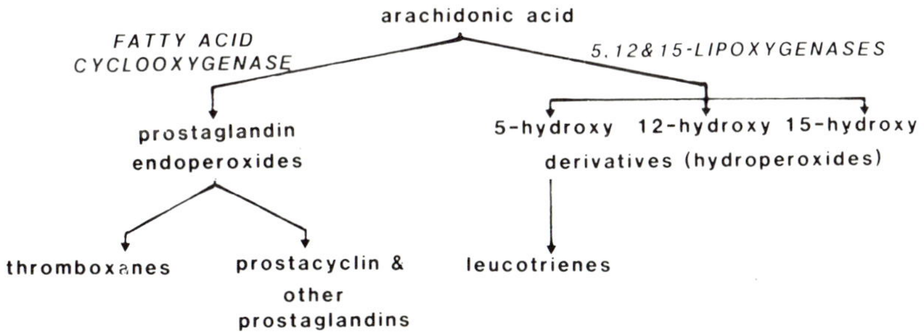

Figure 3.14 Overview of pathways of arachidonic acid metabolism

In the present state of knowledge, it is only the pathway catalysed by the cyclooxygenase (prostaglandin endoperoxide synthetase) that appears relevant to migraine, though this may not remain so as information accumulates. Cyclo-oxygenase appears to be present in all cell membranes[182]. So far there is no evidence of involvement in migraine of the alternative lipo-oxygenase pathway.

The initial reaction catalysed by cyclo-oxygenase converts arachidonic acid to the prostaglandin endoperoxide PGG_2 which is then reduced to PGH_2 (Figure 3.15).

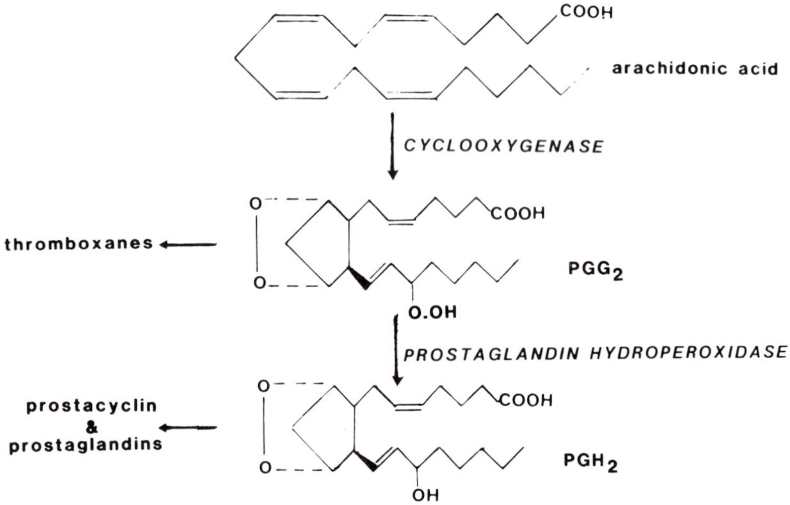

Figure 3.15 Formation of prostaglandin endoperoxides

The endoperoxide PGG_2 gives rise to the thromboxanes (Figure 3.16), the non-enzymatic hydrolysis of thromboxane A_2 proceeding rapidly under physiological conditions.

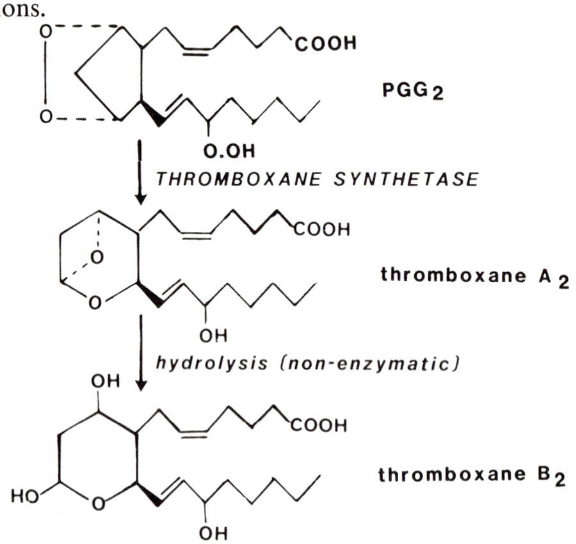

Figure 3.16 Thromboxane formation from protaglandin endoperoxide PGG_2

Thromboxanes are found in platelets, leukocytes, the lungs and the spleen[182]. The endoperoxide PGH_2 is converted to prostacyclin (PGI_2) or to prostaglandins of the D_2, E_2 and F_2 series (Figure 3.17).

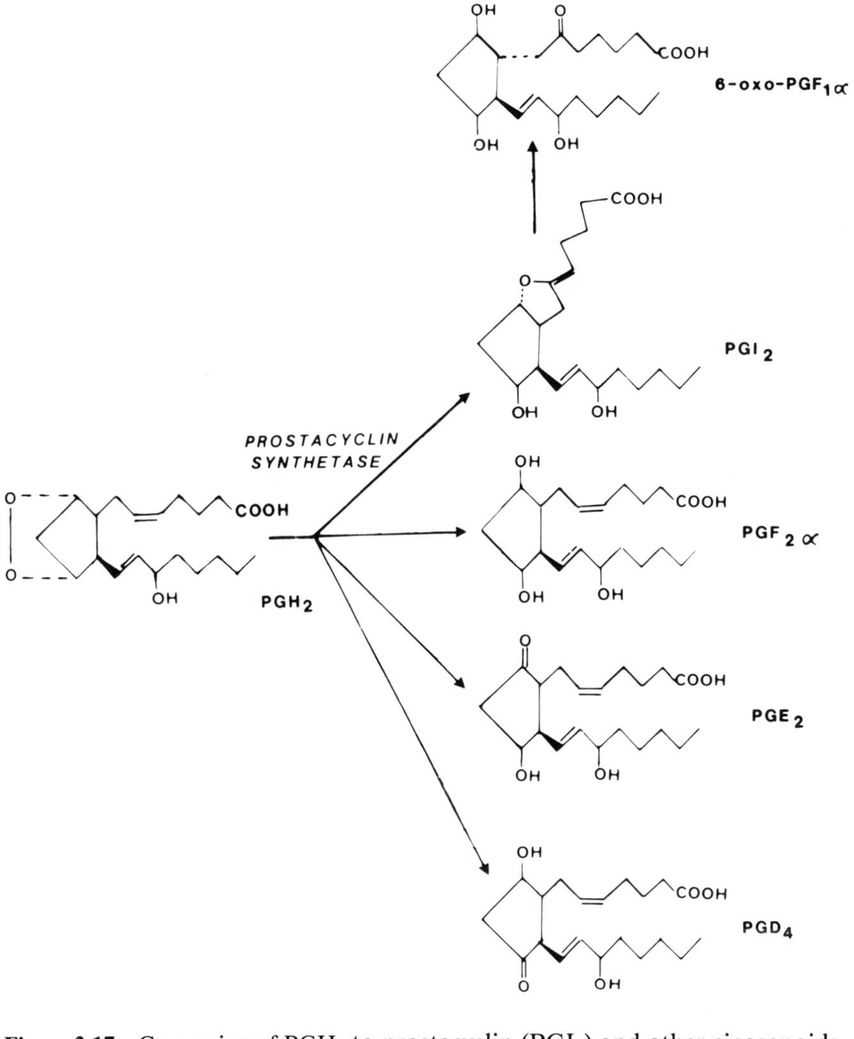

Figure 3.17 Conversion of PGH_2 to prostacyclin (PGI_2) and other eicosanoids

3.6.1.2 Metabolism

The foregoing discussion of eicosanoid synthesis has, for simplicity, indicated the pathways of formation of only some of these compounds. From the point of view of vascular and platelet function the important eicosanoids are, respectively, prostacyclin (PGI_2) and thromboxane A_2 (TxA_2). Only the metabolism of these two eicosanoids will be discussed in this section.

Figure 3.18 shows the conversion of prostacyclin (PGI_2) to the stable compound 6-oxo (or keto) – $PGF_{1\alpha}$. This conversion is a hydrolytic reaction which proceeds under physiological conditions without the agency of enzymatic activity[183]. In liver, blood vessels and the kidneys, the 6-oxo-$PGF_{1\alpha}$, and prostacyclin, undergo further metabolic degradation. Wong *et al.*[184] have proposed a scheme for these additional metabolic pathways in the liver, much as shown in Figure 3.18. Detailed information about the metabolic disposition of prostacyclin in humans is now available[185].

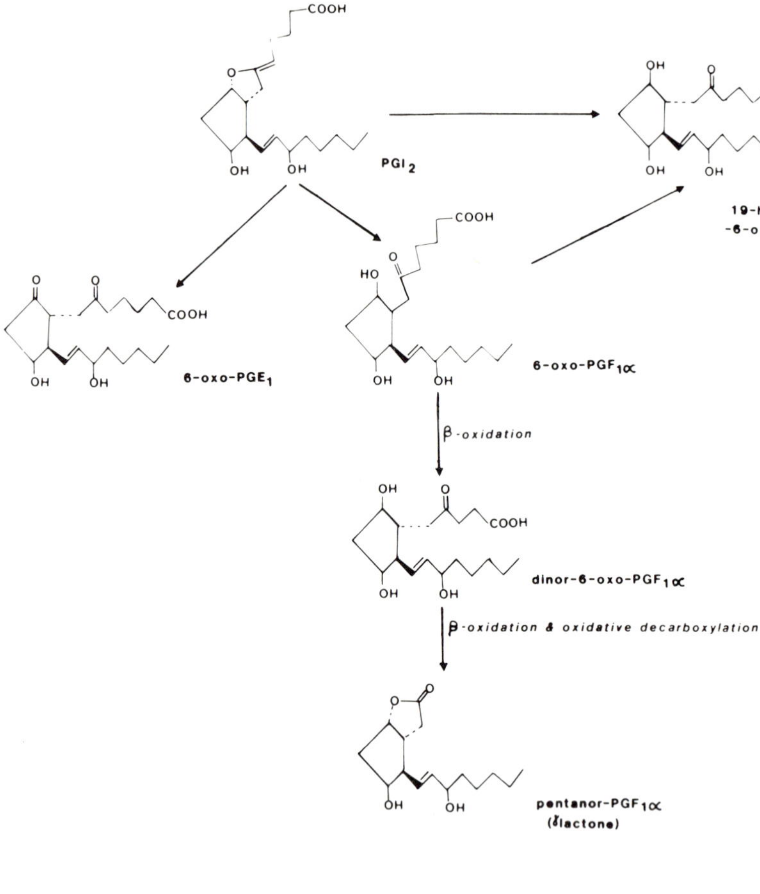

Figure 3.18 Pathways of prostacyclin metabolism

In man, the major metabolite of thromboxane A_2 in urine is 2,3- dinor-TxB_2. This results from fatty acid oxidation of thromboxane B_2, the stable, biologically inactive, immediate metabolite of thromboxane A_2 (Figure 3.19).

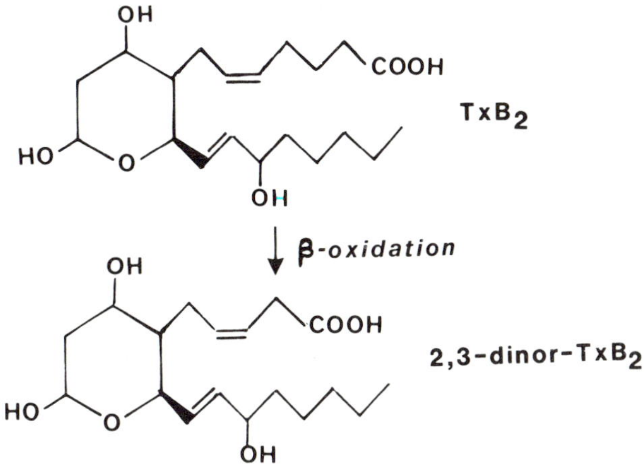

Figure 3.19 Oxidation of thromboxane B_2

Many eicosanoids, but not prostacyclin, are metabolised in the lungs[183] as well as in the other sites mentioned above.

3.6.1.3 Occurrence

The various eicosanoids occur ubiquitously in the animal body. In the present context interest lies mainly in their occurrence in platelets (and perhaps in leukocytes) and in vascular endothelium. In platelets the thromboxane pathway is well developed to the exclusion of the pathway to prostaglandin formation. In vascular endothelium, including that of the cerebral arteries[186], the preferred direction of cyclo-oxygenase activity is towards prostaglandin synthesis. Moncada and Vane[182] have suggested a possible mechanism of interaction between the platelet and the endothelial cell eicosanoid pathways (Figure 3.20). Platelet activation and aggregation is associated with prostaglandin endoperoxide and thromboxane formation. It is suggested that when aggregating platelets come in contact with endothelium the prostaglandin endoperoxides formed within platelets can leak into plasma and from there be taken up by endothelial cells. Within these cells they serve as substrates for prostacyclin rather than thromboxane formation. When this prostacyclin is released and comes in contact with platelets it inhibits further platelet aggregation. Thus healthy endothelium would possess antithrombotic and platelet antiaggregatory mechanisms activated by the beginnings of platelet aggregation and endoperoxide synthesis.

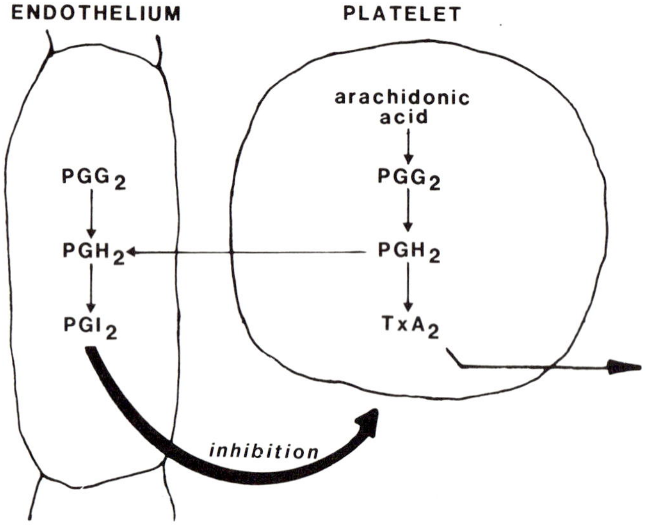

Figure 3.20 The suggested relationship between endothelial and platelet eicosanoids.

The vascular-active eicosanoids TxA_2 and PGI_2 have transient existences, both being inactivated by non-enzymatic hydrolysis. Their half lives, after formation, are of the order of 30 seconds in the case of thromboxane A_2, and of 2–3 minutes in the case of prostacyclin. Both substances are nearly always measured in biological materials in terms of the concentrations of their hydrolysis products (thromboxane B_2 in the case of thromboxane A_2, and 6-oxo-$PGF_{1\alpha}$ in the case of prostacyclin). However the urinary di-nor-metabolites and other β-oxidation derivatives of the hydrolysis products may represent a better measure of turnover of the two eicosanoids. The precursor endoperoxides PGG_2 and PGH_2 have half lives of approximately 5 minutes only.

In relation to the pathogenesis of migraine it may be worth noting that as little as 5 minutes of brain ischaemia in gerbils produces an approximate tenfold increase in the cerebral $PGF_{2\alpha}$ and 6-oxo-$PGF_{2\alpha}$ contents[187].

3.6.1.4 Effects

Thromboxane A_2, the different prostaglandins, the leukotrienes and probably the prostaglandin endoperoxides have a variety of known actions in different tissues, and probably some as yet undiscovered ones. In the present text only the effects of the eicosanoids on platelet and vascular wall function, and on pain production, will be considered.

Thromboxane A_2 Thromboxane A_2 is a potent platelet aggregating agent and constrictor of vascular smooth muscle. Thromboxane A_2 acts by inhibiting platelet adenylate cyclase, thus reducing levels of cAMP in platelets. Wolfe[188] stated that thromboxane A_2 constricted large and small intracranial vessels and decreased cerebral blood flow.

Prostacyclin The actions of prostacyclin are in general the converse of those of thromboxane A_2. It is a powerful vasodilator (including dilatation of cerebral arteries,[189,190] and a potent platelet antiaggregatory agent (even at concentrations as low as 1 $\mu g/l$). Burnstock[34] stated that high doses of prostacyclin have a vasoconstrictor effect. Infused intravenously into man, prostacyclin causes a fall in diastolic blood pressure, presumably resulting from vasodilatation, and facial flushing; mean cerebral blood flow is reduced[191]. Prostacyclin applied directly to pial vessels causes dilatation and increased blood flow, with changed cerebral glucose utilisation. Given intravenously, prostacyclin does not alter cephalic arterio-venous blood shunting in rabbits[192]. Brandt *et al.*[193] regarded the available evidence as suggesting that prostacyclin had the function of maintaining cerebral vascular tone. Prostacyclin causes renin release. It also stimulates platelet adenylate cyclase, thus raising cAMP levels.

The prostacyclin metabolite 6-oxo-$PGF_{1\alpha}$ appears to lack many of the vasodilating properties of prostacyclin[190].

Endoperoxides There is evidence that the prostaglandin endoperoxides have some capacity to facilitate platelet aggregation in their own rights[194]. The endoperoxides reduce cAMP concentrations. PGH_2 causes contraction of isolated arteries[189].

Other prostaglandins Although early studies suggested prostaglandins of the E and F series were vasoactive, much of this work needs to be reassessed in view of the subsequent discoveries of the highly potent agents thromboxane A_2 and prostacyclin. Carlson *et al.*[194] found that intravenous PGE_1 caused cutaneous flushing and headache, with cramping abdominal pain and soreness of the legs. Pickard *et al.*[195] and Wolfe[196] stated that prostaglandins $PGF_{2\alpha}$ and PGE_2 constricted large and small intracranial vessels and reduced the cerebral blood flow. Prostaglandin PGE_2 dilates the external carotid tree, and causes increased extracranial and skin blood flow[197].

Prostaglandins PGD_2 and PGE_1 inhibit platelet aggregation[198]. Certain prostaglandins, e.g. PGE_2 seem capable of inducing pain, perhaps when they are present together with algesic substances such as bradykinin[182]. The actual prostaglandins responsible for this pain-producing effect remain unclear.

3.6.2 Eicosanoid changes in migraine

The opposing vascular and platelet effects of thromboxane A_2 and prostacyclin might be seen as possible explanations, or at least as possible contributory components, for the vascular events of migraine. Wolfe[188] discussed the possible role of eicosanoids in migraine, without providing any direct observational evidence for the possibilities he canvassed. Parantainen and Vapaatalo[199] stated that there have been either inconsistent findings or no changes in plasma prostacyclin, thromboxane A_2, thromboxane B_2, 6-oxo-$PGF_{1\alpha}$, PGE_1 or PGE_2 levels in migraine. Anthony[200] found no change in circulating levels of prostaglandin PGE_1 during migraine attacks, but Amroyan[201] reported raised levels of this eicosanoid during attacks. Vardi *et al.*[202] found increased salivary levels of PGE_2 in six patients during migraine attacks. We have traced no measurements of eicosanoid turnover in migraine.

Peatfield *et al.*[191,203] infused prostacyclin intravenously into eight migraine and eight cluster headache sufferers. The prostacyclin dose was sufficient to induce marked flushing, and induced mild throbbing headache in the majority, but no instances of the patients' typical headaches occurred. Parantainen and Vapaatalo[199] stated that PGE_1 infusion may cause pulsatile headaches, sometimes unilateral and sometimes with prior visual disturbance.

3.6.3 Interpretation of eicosanoid changes in migraine

The increased platelet aggregation that occurs before and during migraine attacks might be expected to be associated with thromboxane A_2 synthesis in platelets, and with the subsequent release of this eicosanoid into plasma. Released thromboxane A_2 might cause vasoconstriction. If the constriction was severe enough in the cerebral and scalp circulations, ischaemic endothelial injury might activate the prostaglandin cascade mechanism in endothelial cells, leading to prostacyclin synthesis and release into the circulation[204]. This released prostacyclin might tend to terminate the platelet aggregation–thromboxane synthesis cycle, and at the same time initiate the vasodilatation phase of migraine. Such a scenario suggests a mechanism for active vasodilatation in the disorder, which seems a more satisfactory explanation for this phenomenon than the mere absence of a degree of tonic contraction maintained by circulating serotonin. However, such a postulated series of events does not explain why the vasoconstrictive and vasodilating events of migraine have a quite restricted rather than a generalised distribution in the body. There is, as yet, no experimental evidence to support the suggested hypothesis. Such evidence might, in fact, be difficult to obtain, particularly if eicosanoid changes occurred mainly in the cerebral circulation (for some as yet unknown reason). Thromboxane A_2 and prostacyclin have transient existences in the circulation, and the former can be metabolically degraded in the lungs. Therefore it would probably be necessary to measure these eicosanoids in jugular venous blood from the affected side of the head to detect relevant changes in their intravascular levels during migraine attacks. Changes in circulating or urinary levels of metabolites of thromboxane A_2 and prostacyclin might not be large enough to be detected unequivocably if the changes in production of the eicosanoids were restricted to the head.

The failure of Peatfield *et al.*[191,203] to mimic migraine and cluster headache in predisposed persons by infusing prostacyclin is not necessarily evidence against the suggested mechanism. It may be that prior exposure to thromboxane A_2 activity is necessary before prostacyclin can produce migraine headache in those with a tendency to the disorder.

Parantainen and Vapaatalo[199] tentatively suggested that the initial arterial spasm of migraine may be due to prostaglandin E, with this eicosanoid and prostacyclin then causing opening of arterio-venous shunts, vasodilatation and pain sensitisation.

Thus while there is so far very little experimental evidence to support the possibility that eicosanoids play a role in the migraine mechanism, they have up to the present scarcely been the subject of adequate investigation in the disorder. Their properties certainly make them attractive candidates for a role in migraine pathogenesis.

References

1. Smith, I., Francis, P.L. and Mullen, P.E. (1981). Pineal hormones and man. In Rose, F.C. (ed.). *Metabolic Disorders of the Nervous System,* London: Pitman, 49–61
2. Da Prada, M. and Pletscher, A. (1972). Uptake, metabolism, storage and release of 5-hydroxytryptamine in blood platelets. *Research and Clinical Studies in Headache,* **3,** 202–213
3. Da Prada, M., Richards, J.G. and Ketti, R. (1981). Amine storage organelles in platelets, in Gordon, J.L. (ed.). *Platelets in Biology and Pathology,* **2,** Amsterdam: Elsevier, 107–145
4. Lingjaerde, O. (1977). Platelet uptake and storage of serotonin. In Essman, W.B. (ed.). *Serotonin in Health and Disease.* Vol. 4. New York: Spectrum, 139–199
5. Salmon, S.,Bonciani, M., Fanciullacci, M., Marianelli, L., Michelacci, S. and Sicuteri, F. (1982). A putative 5-HT control feedback in migraine and cluster headache attacks. In Critchley, M., Friedman, A.P., Gorini, S. and Sicuteri, F. (eds.) Headache: Physiopathological and Clinical Concepts. *Advances in Neurology,* **33,** 265–274
6. Launay, J.M., Lemaitre, B.J., Husson, H.P., Dreux, C., Hartmann, L. and Da Prada, M. (1982). Melatonin synthesis by rabbit platelets. *Life Sciences,* **31,** 1487–1496
7. Vanhoutte, P.M. (1983). Introductory remarks: why 5-hydroxytryptamine? *Federation Proceedings,* **42,** 211–212
8. Parbtani, A. and Stewart Cameron, J. (1978). Platelets, serotonin, and immune-complex disease. *Lancet,* **2,** 679
9. Janssen, P.A.J. (1983). 5-HT_2 receptor blockade to study serotonin-induced pathology. *Trends in Pharmacological Sciences,* **4,** 198–206
10. Peroutka, S.J. and Snyder, S.H. (1983). Multiple serotonin receptors and their physiological significance. *Federation Proceedings,* **42,** 213–217
11. Humphrey, P.P.A., Feniuk, W. and Watts, A.D. (1983). Pre-junctional effects of 5-hydroxytryptamine on noradrenergic nerves in the cardiovascular system. *Federation Proceedings,* **42,** 218–222
12. Haigler, H.J. (1982). Characteristics of extravascular serotonin receptors in the brain. *Advances in Neurology,* **33,** 283–289
13. Armstrong, D. Dry, R.M.L., Keele, C.A. and Markham, J.W. (1952). Pain-producing actions of tryptamine and 5-hydroxytryptamine. *Journal of Physiology (London),* **117,** 70–71
14. Thompson, J.H. (1977). Serotonin (5-hydroxytryptamine)and the alimentary system. In Essman, W.B. *Serotonin in Health and Disease, Vol. 4,* New York: Spectrum, 201–392.
15. Bulbring, E. and Crema, A. (1958). Observations concerning the action of 5-hydroxytryptamine on the peristaltic reflex. *British Journal of Pharmacology,* **13,** 444–457
16. Bulbring, E. and Lin, R.C.Y. (1958). The effect of intraluminal application of 5-hydroxytryptamine and 5-hydroxytryptophan on peristalsis: the local production of 5-HT and its release in relation to intraluminal pressure and propulsive activity. *Journal of Physiology,* **140,** 381–407
17. Kosterlitz, H.W. and Robinson, J.A. (1957). Inhibition of the peristaltic reflex of the isolated guinea-pig ileum. *Journal of Physiology,* **136,** 249–262
18. Costa, M. and Furness, J.B. (1979). On the possibility that an indoleamine is a neurotransmitter in the gastrointestinal tract. *Biochemical Pharmacology,* **28,** 565–571
19. Vanhoutte, P.M. and Cohen, R.A. (1983). The elusory role of serotonin in vascular function and disease. *Biochemical Pharmacology,* **32,** 3671–3674
20. Ostergaard, J.R., Mikkelsen, E. and Voldby, B. (1981). Effects of 5-hydroxytryptamine and ergotamine on human superficial temporal artery. *Cephalalgia,* **1,** 223–228
21. Hardebo, J.E., Edvinsson, L., Owman, C.H. and Svendgaard, N.A. (1978). Potentiation and antagonism of serotonin effects on intracranial and extracranial vessels. Possible implications in migraine. *Neurology,* **28,** 64–70

22. Saxena, P.R. (1972). The effects of antimigraine drugs on the vascular responses by 5-hydroxytryptamine and related biogenic substances on the external carotid bed of dogs: possible pharmacological implications to their antimigraine action. *Headache,* **12,** 44–54
23. Muller-Schweinitzer, E. and Fanchamps, A. (1982). Effects on arterial receptors of ergot derivatives used in migraine. In Critchley, M. Friedman, A.P., Gorini, S. and Sicuteri, F. (eds.) Headache: Physiopathological and Clinical Concepts. *Advances in Neurology,* **33,** 343–356
24. Van Nueten, J.M. (1983). 5-Hydroxytryptamine and precapillary vessels. *Federation Proceedings,* **42,** 223–227
25. Edvinsson, L. and MacKenzie, E.T. (1977). Amine mechanisms in the cerebral circulation. *Pharmacolgical Reviews,* **28,** 275–348
26. Pickard, J.D., Mackenzie, E.T. and Harper, A.M. (1978). Serotonin and prostaglandins: intracranial and extracranial effects with reference to migraine. In Greene, R. (ed.). *Current Concepts in Migraine Research.* New York: Raven Press, 101–104
27. Grimson, B.S., Robinson, S.C., Danford, E.T., Tindall, G.T. and Greenfield, J.C. Jr. (1969). Effect of serotonin on internal and external carotid artery blood flow in the baboon. *American Journal of Physiology,* **216,** 50–55
28. Deshmukh, V.D. and Harper, A.M. (1973). The effect of serotonin on cerebral and extracerebral blood flow with possible implications in migraine. *Acta Neurologica Scandinavica,* **49,** 649–658
29. Edvinsson, L. and Hardebo, J-E. (1978). Receptors for 5-hydroxytryptamine in intracranial and extracranial arteries of cat and man. In Greene, R. (ed.). *Current Concepts in Migraine Research,* New York: Raven Press, 141–147
30. Welch, K.M.A., Spira, P.J., Knowles, L. and Lance, J.W. (1974). Simultaneous measurement of internal and external carotid blood flow in the monkey. *Neurology,* **24,** 450–457
31. Lance, J.W., Spira, P.J., Mylecharane, E.J., Lord, G.D.A. and Duckworth, J.W. (1978). Evaluation of drugs applicable to treatment of migraine in the cranial circulation of the monkey. *Research and Clinical Studies in Headache,* **6,** 13–18
32. Saxena, P.R. and Tangri, K.K. (1981). Arteriovenous shunting and 5-hydroxytryptamine: possible implications in migraine pathophysiology. *Headache.* **21,** 125
33. Saxena, P.R. (1982). Agonists and antagonists of vascular receptors. *Advances in Neurology.* **33,** 309–314
34. Burnstock, G. (1981). Nervous control of cerebral blood vessels: a new hypothesis for the mechanisms underlying migraine. In Rose, F.C. and Zilkha, K.J. (eds.). *Progress in Migraine Research,* **1,** London: Pitman, 17–32
35. Olesen, J. and Skinhoj, E. (1971). The influence of certain vasoactive amines on the regional cerebral blood flow in man. *Proceedings of the International Headache Symposium, Elsinore, Denmark.* Basel: Sandoz, 145–152
36. Lance, J.W. Anthony, M. and Gonski, A. (1967). Serotonin, the carotid body and cranial vessels in migraine. *Archives of Neurology,* **16,** 553–558
37. Olesen, J. (1981). Effect of serotonin on regional cerebral blood flow (rCBF) in man. *Cephalalgia,* **1,** 7–10
38. Peltola, P. (1972). Bradykinin induced release of serotonin in man. *Research and Clinical Studies in Headache,* **3,** 299–303
39. DeClerck, F.F. and Herman, A.G. (1983). 5-Hydroxytryptamine and platelet aggregation. *Fedèration Proceedings,* **42,** 228–232
40. Arendt, J. (1981). Melatonin (? neurohormone). In Rose, F.C. (ed.). *Metabolic Disorders of the Nervous System,* London: Pitman, 40–48
41. Leach, C.M. and Thorburn, G.D. (1980). A comparison of the inhibitory effects of melatonin and indomethacin on platelet aggregation and thromboxane release. *Prostaglandins,* **20,** 51–56
42. Forster, C. and Whalley, E.T. (1981). Comparison of the contraction produced by various tryptamine analogues on human basilar arterial and rat aortic strips in vitro. *Cephalalgia,* **1,** 217–221
43. Sicuteri, F., Testi, A. and Anselmi, B. (1961). Biochemical investigations in headache. Increases in the hydroxyindoleacetic acid excretion during migraine attacks. *International Archives of Allergy,* **19,** 55–58
44. Curran, D.A., Hinterberger, H. and Lance, J.W. (1965). Total plasma serotonin, 5-hydroxyindoleacetic acid and p-hydroxy-m-methoxy mandelic acid excretion in normal and

migrainous subjects. *Brain,* **88,** 997–1010

45. Curzon, G. Barrie, M. and Wilkinson, M.I.P. (1969). Relationships between headache and amine changes after administration of reserpine to migrainous patients. *Journal of Neurology, Neurosurgery and Psychiatry,* **32,** 555–561
46. Deanovic, Z., Iskric, S. and Dupelj, M. (1975). Fluctuation of 5-hydroxyindole compounds in the urine of migrainous patients. *Biomedicine,* **23,** 346–349
47. Mück-Šeler, D., Deanovic, Z. and Dupelj, M. (1982). Serotonin-releasing factors in migrainous patients. *Advances in Neurology,* **33,** 257–264
48. Blau, J.N., Horsfield,D., Quick, J. and Cumings, J.N. (1967). The production of migraine and biochemical changes in induced attacks. In Smith, R. (ed.). *Background to Migraine,* London: Heinemann, 146–153
49. Curzon, G., Theaker, P. and Phillips, B. (1966). Excretion of 5-hydroxyindolyl acetic acid (5-HIAA) in migraine. *Journal of Neurology, Neurosurgery and Psychiatry.* **32,** 555–561
50. Curzon, G. (1967). Amine changes in migraine. In Smith, R. (ed.). *Background to Migraine,* London: Heinemann, 134–143
51. Kangasniemi, P., Sonninen, V. and Rinne, U.K. (1972). Excretion of free and conjugated 5-HIAA and VMA in urine and concentration of 5-HIAA and HVA in CSF during migraine attacks and free intervals. *Heachache,* **12,** 62–65
52. Nattero, G. (1982). Menstrual headache. In Critchley, M., Friedman, A.P., Gorini, S. and Sicuteri, F. (eds.). Headache: Physiopathological and Clinical Concepts. *Advances in Neurology,* **33,** 215–226
53. Anthony, M. and Hinterberger, H. (1975). Amine turnover in migraine. *Proceedings of the Australian Association of Neurologists.* **12,** 43–47
54. Anthony, M. (1972). The mechanisms underlying migraine. *Medical Journal of Australia,* **2,** Special Supplement, 11–15
55. Anthony, M. (1982). Serotonin and cyclic nucleotides in migraine. *Advances in Neurology,* **33,** 45–49
56. Anthony, M., Hinterberger, H. and Lance, J.W. (1967). Plasma serotonin in migraine and stress. *Archives of Neurology,* **16,** 544–552
57. Berstad, J.R. (1976). Total 5-hydroxyindoles in blood related to migraine attacks. *Acta Neurologica Scandinavica.* **54,** 293–300
58. Hilton, B.P. and Cumings, J.N. (1972). 5-Hydroxytryptamine levels and platelet aggregation responses in subjects with acute migraine headaches. *Journal of Neurology, Neurosurgery and Psychiatry,* **35,** 505–509
59. Hinterberger, H., Anthony, M. and Vagholkar, M.K. (1968). Platelet 5-hydroxytryptamine and adenine nucleotides, serum-arginylesterase and plasma 11-hydroxycorticosteroids in migraine. *Clinical Science,* **34,** 271–276
60. Mück-Šeler, D., Deanovic, Z. and Dupelj, M. (1979). Platelet serotonin (5-HT) and 5-HT releasing factor in plasma of migrainous patients. *Headache,* **19,** 14–17
61. Rydzevsky, W. (1976). Serotonin (5-HT) in migraine: levels in whole blood in and between attacks. *Headache,* **16,** 16–19
62. D'Andrea, G., Toldo, M., Cortelazzo, S. and Milone, F.F. (1982). Platelet activity in migraine. *Headache,* **22,** 207–212
63. Sjaastad, O. (1975). The significance of blood serotonin levels in migraine. A critical review. *Acta Neurologica Scandinavica,* **51,** 200–210
64. Sjaastad, O. (1975). Vascular and biochemical changes in migraine. In Saxena, P.R. (ed.). *Migraine and Related Headache.* Uden: Sandoz, 55–69
65. Somerville, B.W. (1976). Platelet-bound and free serotonin levels in jugular and forearm venous blood during migraine. *Neurology,* **28,** 41–45
66. Salmon, S., Bonciani, M., Fanciullacci, M., Marianelli, L., Michelacci, S. and Sicuteri, F. (1982). A putative 5-HT central feedback in migraine and cluster headache attacks. *Advances in Neurology,* **33,** 265–274
67. Hyppa, M.T. and Kangasnemi, P. (1977). Variation of plasma free tryptophane and CSF 5-HIAA during migraine. *Headache,* **17,** 25–27
68. Salmon, S., Fanciullacci, M., Bonciani, M. and Sicuteri, F. (1978). Plasma tryptophan in migraine. *Headache,* **17,** 238–241
69. Anselmi, B., Baldi, E., Casacci, F. and Salmon, S. (1980). Endogenous opioids in cerebrospinal fluid and blood in idiopathic headache sufferers. *Headache,* **20,** 294–299

70. Anthony, M., Hinterberger, H. and Lance, J.W. (1968). Studies of serotonin metabolism in migraine. *Proceedings of the Australian Association of Neurologists,* **5,** 109–112
71. Dalsgaard-Nielsen, T. and Genefke, I.K. (1974). Serotonin (5-hydroxy-tryptamine) release and uptake in platelets from healthy persons and migrainous patients in attack-free intervals. *Headache,* **14,** 26–32
72. Carroll, J.D., Coppen, A., Swade, C.C., and Wood, K.M. (1980). Blood platelet 5-hydroxytryptamine accumulation and migraine. *Upsala Journal of Medical Science,* Supplement 31, 10–12
73. Carroll, J.D., Coppen, A., Swade, C.C. and Wood, K.M. (1982). Blood platelet 5-hydroxytryptamine accumulation and migraine. *Advances in Neurology,* **33,** 233–235
74. Coppen, A., Swade, C., Wood, K. and Carroll, J.D. (1979). Platelet 5-hydroxytryptamine accumulation and migraine. *Lancet,* **2,** 914
75. Malmgren, R., Olsson, P., Tornling, G. and Unge, G. (1978). Acetylsalicylic asthma and migraine. A defect in serotonin (5HT) uptake in platelets. *Thrombosis Research,* **13,** 1137–1139
76. Malmgren, R., Olsson, P., Tornling, G. and Unge, G. (1979). Migraine, a platelet disorder. *Lancet,* **2,** 1198
77. Hanington, E., Jones, R.J., Amess, J.A.L. and Wachowicz, P. (1981). Migraine: a platelet disorder. *Lancet,* **2,** 720–723
78. Malmgren, R., Olsson, P., Tornling, G. and Unge, G. (1980). The 5-hydroxytryptamine take-up mechanism in normal platelets and platelets from migraine and asthmatic patients. *Thrombosis Research,* **18,** 733–742
79. Launay, J.M., Pradalier, A., Dreux, C. and Dry, J. (1982). Platelet serotonin uptake and migraine. *Cephalalgia,* **2,** 57–59
80. Pradalier, A. and Launay, J.M. (1982). 5-hydroxytryptamine uptake by platelets from migrainous patients. *Lancet,* **1,** 862
81. Lance, J.W. Anthony, M. and Hinterberger, H. (1970). Migraine and 5-hydroxytryptamine. In Cochrane, A.L. (ed.). *Background to Migraine.* London: Heinemann, 155–161
82. Anthony, M. and Lance, J.W. (1975). The role of serotonin. In Pearce, J. (ed.). *Modern Topics in Migraine.* London: Heinemann, 107–123
83. Dvilansky, A., Rishpon, S., Nathan, I., Zolatow, Z. and Dorczyn, A.D. (1976). Release of platelet 5-hydroxytryptamine by plasma taken from patients during and between migraine attack. *Pain,* **2,** 315–318
84. Skarby, T., Tfelt-Hansen, P., Gjerris, F., Edvinsson, L. and Olesen, J. (1982). Characterization of 5-hydroxytryptamine receptors in human temporal arteries: comparison betrween migraine sufferers and nonsufferers. *Annals of Neurology,* **12,** 272–277
85. Sicuteri, F. (1973). 5-hydroxytryptamine supersensitivity as a new theory of essential headache. In Cumings, J.N. (ed.). *Background to Migraine.* London: Heinemann, 45–56
86. Botney, M. (1981). An inquiry into the genesis of migraine headache. *Headache,* **21,** 179–185
87. Welch, K.M.A., Gaudet, R., Wang, T.P.F. and Chabi, E. (1977). Transient cerebral ischemia and brain serotonin: relevance to migraine. *Headache,* **17,** 145–147
88. Crook, M. (1981). Migraine: a biochemical headache? *Biochemical Society Transactions,* **9,** 351–357
89. Papavasaliou, P.S., Cotzias, G.C., Duby, S.E., Steck, A.J., Bell, M. and Lawrence, W.H. (1972). Melatonin and Parkinsonism. *Journal of the American Medical Association,* **221,** 88–89
90. Behar, A.J., Deutsch, E., Pomerantz, E., Pfeifer, Y. and Sulman, F.G. (1979). Serotonin and the carotid body. *Lancet,* **1,** 550
91. Kimball, R.W., Friedman, A.P. and Vallejo, E. (1960). Effect of serotonin in migraine patients. *Neurology,* **10,** 107–111
92. Sandler, M. (1975). Monoamines and migraine: a path through the wood, in Diamond, S., Dalessio, D.J., Graham, J.R. and Medina, J.L. (eds.). *Vasoactive Substances Relevant to Migraine.* Springfield, Ill.: C. C. Thomas, 3–18
93. Damasio, H. and Beck, D. (1978). Migraine, thrombocytopenia, and serotonin metabolism. *Lancet,* **1,** 240–242
94. Heyck, H. (1970). The importance of arterio-venous shunts in the pathogenesis of migraine. In Cochrane, A.L. (ed.). *Background to Migraine.* London: Heinemann. 19–25
95. Bruyn, G.W. (1982). Cerebral cortex and migraine. *Advances in Neurology,* **33,** 151–169

96. Willoughby, J.O. (1981). The pathophysiology of vegetative symptoms in migraine. *Lancet,* **2,** 445 – 446
97. De Met, E.M. and Halaris, A.E. (1979). Origin and distribution of 3-methoxy-4-hydroxyphenylglycol in body fluids. *Biochemical Pharmacology,* **28,** 3043 – 3050
98. Jenner, P. and Marsden, C.D. (1982). Interpretation of radioactive ligand binding to cerebral dopamine receptors. In Marsden, C.D. and Fahn, S. (eds.). *Movement Disorders.* London: Butterworth, 356 – 368
99. Wang P-C., Kuchel, O., Buu, N.T. and Genest, J. (1983). Catecholamine glucuronidation: an important metabolic pathway for dopamine in the rat. *Journal of Neurochemistry,* **40,** 1435 – 1440
100. Van Loon, G.R. and Sole, M.J. (1980). Plasma dopamine: source, regulation and significance. *Metabolism,* **29,** 1119 – 1123
101. Mefford, I.N., Ward, M.M., Miles, L., Taylor, B., Chesney, M.A., Keegan, D.l. and Barchas, J.D. (1981). III. Determination of plasma catecholamine and free 3,4-dihydroxyphenylacetic acid in continuously collected human plasma by high performance liquid chromatography with electrochemical detection. *Life Sciences,* **28,** 477 – 483
102. Robertson, D., Johnson, G. A. Robertson, R.M., Nies, A.S., Shand, D.G. and Oates, J.A. (1979). Comparative assessment of stimuli that release neuronal and adrenomedullary catecholamines in man. *Circulation,* **59,** 637 – 643
103. Bravo, E.L. and Tarazi, R.C. (1982). Plasma catecholamines in clinical investigation: a useful index or a meaningless number. *Journal of Laboratory and Clinical Medicine.* **100,** 155 – 160
104. Goldstein, D.S., Feuerstein, G., Izzo, J.L.Jr., Kopin, I.J. and Keiser, H.R. (1981) II. Validity and reliability of liquid chromatography with electochemical detection for measuring plasma levels of norepinephrine and epinephrine in man. *Life Sciences,* **28,** 467 – 475
105. Hoffbrand, B.I. and Forsyth, R.P. (1973). Regional blood flow changes during norepinephrine, tyramine and methoxamine infusions in the unanaesthesized rhesus monkey. *Journal of Pharmacology and Experimental Therapeutics,* **184,** 656 – 661
106 Cahen, R.L. (1972). Emetic effect of biogenic amines. *Research and Clinical Studies in Headache,* **3,** 227 – 244
107. Goldberg, L.I. (1975). The dopamine vascular receptor. *Biochemical Pharmacology,* **24,** 651 – 653
108. Von Essen, C., Zervas, N.T., Brown, D.R., Koltun, W.A. and Pickren, K.S. (1980). Local cerebral blood flow in the dog during intravenous infusion of dopamine. *Surgical Neurology,* **13,** 181 – 187
109. Scrutton, M.C. and Wallis, R.B. (1981). Catecholamine receptors. In Gordon, J.L. (ed.). *Platelets in Biology and Pathology, 2.* Amsterdam: Elsevier, 179 – 209
110. Hsu, L.K.G., Crisp, A.H., Kalucy, R.S., Koval, R.S., Chen, C.N., Carruthers, M. and Zilkha, K.J. (1977). Early morning migraine. Nocturnal plasma levels of catecholamine, tryptophan, glucose and free fatty acids and sleep encephalographs. *Lancet,* **1,** 447 – 451
111. Hsu,L.K.J., Crisp, A.H., Kalucy, R.S., Koval, J., Chen, C.N., Carruthers, M. and Zilkha, K.J. (1978). Nocturnal plasma levels of catecholamines, tryptophan, glucose, and free fatty acids and the sleeping electroencephalographs of subjects experiencing early morning migraine. In Greene, R. (ed.). *Current Concepts in Migraine Research.* New York: Raven Press, 121 – 130
112. Fog-Moller, F., Genefke, I.K. and Bryndum, B. (1978). Changes in the concentration of catecholamines in blood during spontaneous migraine attacks and reserpine-induced attacks. In Green, R. (ed.). *Current Concepts in Migraine Research.* New York: Raven Press, 115 – 119
113. Anthony, M. (1981). Biochemical indices of sympathetic activity in migraine. *Cephalalgia,* **1,** 83 – 89
114. Sicuteri, F., Boccuni, M. Fanciullacci, M., D'Egidio, P. and Bonciani, M. (1982). A new nonvascular interpretation of syncopal migraine. *Advances in Neurology,* **33,** 199 – 208
115. Kangasniemi, P., Riekkinen, P. and Rinne, U.K. (1979). Kallikrein-like esterase and peptidase activities in CSF during migraine attacks and free intervals. *Headache,* **12,** 66 – 68
116. Wolff, H.G. (1963). *Headache and Other Head Pain.* New York: Oxford University Press, 2nd edition
117. Fowler, C.J., Callingham, B.A., Mantle, T.J. and Tipton, K.F. (1978). Monoamine oxidase A and B: a useful concept? *Biochemical Pharmacology,* **27,** 97 – 101

118. Sandler, M. (1977). Transitory platelet monoamine oxidase deficit in migraine: some reflections. *Headache,* **17,** 153 – 158
119. Bond, P.A. and Cundall, R.L. (1977). Properties of monoamine oxidase (MAO) in human blood platelets, plasma, lymphocytes and granulocytes. *Clinica Chemica Acta,* **80,** 317 – 326
120. Glover, U., Peatfield, R.C., Sandler, M., Zammit-Pace, R., Littlewood, J., Gawel, M.J. and Rose, F.C. (1981). Amine inactivating enzymes in headache patients. In Rose, F.C. and Zilkha, K.J. (eds.). *Progress in Migraine Research, l.* London: Pitman, 95 – 99
121. Collins, G.G.S. and Sandler, M. (1971). Human blood platelet monoamine oxidase. *Biochemical Pharmacology,* **20,** 289 – 296
122. Donnelly, C.H. and Murphy, D.L. (1977). Substrate- and inhibitor-related characteristics of human platelet monoamine oxidase. *Biochemical Pharmacology,* **26,** 853 – 858
123. Bussone, G., Giovannini, P., Boiardi, A. and Boeri, R. (1977). A study of the activity of platelet monoamine oxidase in patients with migraine headaches or with 'cluster' headaches. *European Neurology,* **15,** 157 – 162
124. Belmaker, R.H., Murphy, D.L., Wyatt, R.J. and Loiaux, D.L. (1974). Human platelet monoamine oxidase changes during the menstrual cycle. *Archives of General Psychiatry,* **3l,** 553 – 556
125. Sandler, M., Reveley, M.A. and Glover, V. (1981). Human platelet monoamine oxidase activity in health and disease: a review. *Journal of Clinical Pathology,* **34,** 292 – 302
126. Robinson, D.S., Davis, J.M., Nies, A., Ravaris, C.L. and Sylvester, D. (1971). Relation of sex and aging to monoamine oxidase activity of human brain, plasma and platelets. *Archives of General Psychiatry,* **24,** 536 – 539
127. Gawel, M.J. and Rose, F.C. (1982). Platelet function in migraineurs. In Critchley, M., Friedman, A.P., Gorini, S. and Sicuteri, F. (eds.). Headache-Physiopathological and Clinical Aspects. *Advances in Neurology,* **33,** 237 – 242
128. Peatfield, R.C., Gawel, M.J., Guthrie, D.L., Pearson, T.C., Glover, V., Littlewood, J., Sandler, M. and Rose, F.C. (1982). Platelet size: no correlation with migraine or monoamine oxidase activity. *Journal of Neurology, Neurosurgery and Psychiatry,* **45,** 826 – 829
129. Needham, K., Billett, E., Weil, D., Wicks, M., Russell, S., Hanley, S., Heptinstall, S. and Mayer, R.J. (1981). Platelet monoamine oxidase and platelet properties. In Rose, F.C. and Zilkha, K.J. (eds.). *Progress in Migraine Research, l.* London: Pitman, 53 – 60
130. Peatfield, R., Littlewood, J.T., Glover, V., Sandler, M. and Rose F.C. (1983). Pressure sensitivity to tyramine in patients with headache: relationship to platelet monoamine oxidase and to dietary provocation. *Journal of Neurology, Neurosurgery and Psychiatry,* **46,** 827 – 831
131. Sandler, M. (1978). Implications of the platelet monoamine oxidase deficit during migraine attacks. *Research and Clinical Studies in Headache.* **6,** 65 – 72
132. Sandler, M., Youdim, M.B.H. and Hanington, E. (1974). A phenylethylamine oxidising defect in migraine. *Nature,* **250,** 335 – 337
133. Sicuteri, F., Buffoni, F., Anselmi, B. and Del Bianco, P.L. (1971). Monoamine oxidase activity in migraine and arterial hypertension. *Proceedings of the International Headache Symposium, Elsinore, Denmark.* Basel: Sandoz, 195 – 199
134. Sicuteri, F., Buffoni, F., Anselmi, B. and Del Bianco, P.L. (1972). An enzyme (MAO) defect on the platelets in migraine. *Research and Clinical Studies in Headache,* **3,** 245 – 251
135. Glover, V., Peatfield, R., Zammit-Pace, R., Littlewood, J., Gawel, M., Rose, F.C. and Sandler, M. (1981). Platelet monoamine oxidase activity and headache. *Journal of Neurology, Neurosurgery and Psychiatry,* **44,** 786 – 790
136. Glover, V., Sandler, M., Grant, E., Rose, F.C., Orton, D., Wilkinson, M. and Stevens, D. (1977). Transitory decrease in platelet monamine-oxidase activity during migraine attacks. *Lancet,* **1,** 391 – 393
137. Thomas, D.V. (1982). Platelet monoamine oxidase in migraine. *Advances in Neurology,* **33,** 279 – 281
138. Littlewood, J., Glover, V., Sandler, M., Petty, R., Peatfield, R. and Rose, F.C. (1982). Platelet phenosulphotransferase deficiency in dietary migraine. *Lancet,* **1,** 983 – 986
139. Weinshilboum, R.M., Thoa, N.B., Johnson, D.G., Koplin, I.J. and Axelrod, J. (1971). Proportional release of norepinephrine and dopamine-β-hydroxylase from sympathetic nerves. *Science,* **174,** 1349 – 1351
140. Schanberg, S.M. and Kirshner, N. (1976). Serum dopamine-β-hydroxylase as an indicator of sympathetic activity and primary hypertension. *Biochemical Pharmacology,* **25,**617 – 621

141. Wootten, F.G. and Cardon, P.V. (1973). Plasma dopamine-β-hydroxylase activity. *Archives of Neurology,* **28,** 103–106
142. Gotoh, F., Kanda, T.,Sakai, F., Yamamoto, M. and Takeoka, T., (1976). Serum dopamine-β-hydroxylase activity in migraine. *Archives ofNeurology,* **33,** 656–657
143. Beaven, M.H. (1976). Histamine. *New England Journal of Medicine,* **294,** 30–36;320–325
144. Edvinsson, L., Cervos-Navarro, J., Larsson, L-I., Owman, Ch. and Ronnberg, A.L. (1977). Regional distribution of mast cells containing histamine, dopamine, or 5-hydroxytryptamine in the mammalian brain. *Neurology,* **27,**878–883
145. Schwartz, J-C., Pollard, H. and Quach, T.T. (1980). Histamine as a neurotransmitter in mammalian brain; neurochemical evidence. *Journal of Neurochemistry,* **35,**26–33
146. Barnes, P.J., Ind. P.W. and Brown, M.J. (1982). Plasma histamine and catecholamines in stable asthmatic subjects. *Clinical Science,* **62,** 661–665
147. Huang, M. and Rorstad, O.P. (1983). Effect of vasoactive intestinal peptide, monoamines, prostaglandins and 2-chloro-adenosine on adenylate cyclase in rat cerebral microvessels. *Journal of Neurochemistry,* **40,** 719–726
148. Saxena, P.R. (1978). Arteriovenous shunting and migraine. *Research and Clinical Studies in Headache,* **6,**89–102
149. Swade, C.C., Carroll, J.D. and Coppen, A. (1981). Platelet 5-hydroxytryptamine accumulation in migrainous neuralgia. In Rose, F.C. and Zilkha, K.J. (eds.). *Progress in Migraine Research, l.* London: Pitman, 89–92
150. Pickering, G. W. (1939). Experimental observations on headache. *British Medical Journal,* **1,** 907–912
151. Krabbe, A.A. and Olesen, J. (1982). Effect of histamine on regional cerebral blood flow in man. *Cephalalgia,* **2,** 15–18
152. Sicuteri, F. (1963). Mast cells and their active substances: their role in the pathogenesis of migraine. *Headache,* **3,** 86–92
153. Thonnard-Neumann, E. (1975). Heparin, in Diamond, S., Dalessio, D.J., Graham, J.R. and Medina, J.L. (eds.). *Vasoactive Substances Relevant to Migraine.* Springfield, IU.: Thomas, 67–72
154. Sjaastad, O. and Staastad, O.V. (1970). The histaminuria in vascular headache. *Acta Neurologica Scandinavica,* **46,** 311–342
155. Loisy, C., Arnaud, J.L. and Amelot, A. (1972).Contribution to the study of histamine metabolism in migrainous subjects. *Research and Clinical Studies in Headache,* **3,** 252–259
156. Anthony, M. and Lance, J.W. (1971). Whole blood histamine and plasma serotonin in cluster headache. *Proceedings of the Australian Association of Neurologists,* **8,** 43–46
157. Zimmerman, A.W., Sanders, W.M. and Barlow, M. (1979). Histamine release in migraine. *Neurology,* **29,** 550
158. Sanders, W.M., Zimmerman, A.W., Mahoney, M.A. and Ballow, M. (1980). Leucocyte histamine release in migraine. *Headache,* **20,** 307–310
159. Sicuteri, F. (1976). Migraine, a central biochemical dysnocioception. *Headache,* **16,**145–159
160. Peatfield, R.C. and Rose, F.C. (1981). Ranitidine in migraine. *Annals of Neurology,* **10,** 61
161. Selmaj, K. (1983). Histamine release from leucocytes in migraine. *Cephalalgia,* **3,** 37–40
162. Colman, R.W. (1974). Formation of human plasma kinin. *New England Journal of Medicine,* **291,** 509–515
163. Erdos, E.G. (1976). The kinins. A status report. *Biochemical Pharmacology,* **25,**1563–1569
164. Regoli, D. and Barabe, J. (1980). Pharmacology of bradykinin and related kinin. *Pharmacological Reviews,* **32,** 1–46
165. Goodell, H. (1975). Evolution of the concept of neurokinin in migraine headache. In Diamond, S., Dalessio, D.J., Graham J.R. and Medina, J.L. (eds.). *Vasoactive Substances Relevant to Migraine.* Springfield, Ill: Thomas, 30–33
166. Hulthen, U.L. and Borge, T. (1976). Determination of bradykinin in blood by a sensitive radioimmune assay. *Scandinavian Journal of Clinical Laboratory Investigation,* **36,** 833–839
167. Moskowitz, M.A. and Coughlin, S.R. (1981). Basic properties of the prostaglandins. *Stroke,* **12,** 696–701
168. Robson, J.M. (1967). The effects of drugs on blood vessels, in Smith, R. (ed.) *Background to Migraine. First Migraine Symposium.* London: Heinemann, 117–125
169. Toda, N. (1977). Actions of bradykinin in isolated cerebral and peripheral arteries. *American Journal of Physiology,***232,** H267–H274

170. Sicuteri, F., Fanciullacci, M. and Anselmi, B. (1963). Bradykinin release and inactivation in man. *International Archives of Allergy,* **22,** 77 – 84
171. Keele, C.A. (1967). Polypeptides and other substances which may produce vascular headache. In Smith, R. (ed.). *Background to Migraine. First Migraine Symposium.* London: Heinemann, 126 – 133
172. Streeten, D.H.P., Kerr, L.P., Kerr, C.B., Prior, J.C. and Dalakos, T.G. (1972). Hyperbradykininism:a new orthostatic syndrome. *Lancet,* **2,** 1048 – 1053
173. Sicuteri, F. (1970). Bradykinin and the intracranial circulation in man. *Handbook of Experimental Pharmacology,* **25,**482 – 515
174. Greppi, E. and Sicuteri, F. (1964). *L'Emicrania.* Rome: Edizioni L. Pozzia, cited by Keele, C.A. (1967).loc.cit
175. Chapman, L.F. and Wolff, H.G. (1959). Studies of protedytic enzymes in cerebrospinal fluid: capacity of incubated mixtures of cerebrospinal fluid and plasma proteins to form vasodilator substances that contract the isolated rat uterus. *Archives of Internal Medicine,* **103,**86 – 94
176. Kangasniemi, P., Riekkinen, P.,Penttinen, R., Ivaska, K. and Rinne, U.K. (1974). Enzyme changes in the cerebro-spinal fluid and serum and their correlation to the breakdown of bradykinin during different stages of headache attacks of migraine patients. *Headache,***14,** 139 – 148
177. Elkind, A.H., Friedman, A.P. and Grossman, J. (1964). Cutaneous blood flow in vascular headache of the migraine type. *Neurology,* **14,** 24 – 30
178. Friedman, A.P. (1968). Migraine. Pathophysiology and pathogenesis, in Vinken, P.J. and Bruyn, G.W. (eds.). *Handbook of Clinical Neurology,* **5,** 37 – 44
179. Chapman, L.F., Ramos, A.O., Goodell, H., Silverman, G. and Wolff, H.G.(1960). A humoral agent implicated in vascular headache of the migraine type. *Archives of Neurology,* **3,** 223 – 229
180. Chapman, L.F., Ramos, A.O., Goodell, H. and Wolff, H.G.(1961). Neurohumoral features of afferent fibres in man. Their role in vasodilatation, inflammation and pain. *Archives of Neurology and Phychiatry,* **4,** 617 – 650
181. Wolfe, L.S. (1982). Eicosanoids: prostaglandins, thromboxanes, leukotrienes, and other derivatives of carbon-20 unsaturated fatty acids. *Journal of Neurochemistry,* **38,** 1 – 14
182. Moncada, S. and Vane, J.R. (1979). Arachidonic acid metabolites and the interaction between platelets and blood-vessel walls. *New England Journal of Medicine,* **300,**1142 – 1147
183. Moncada, S. and Vane, J.R. (1979). The role of prostacyclin in vascular tissue. *Federation Proceedings,* **38,** 66 – 71
184. Wong, P.Y-K., Lee, W.H., Quilley, C.P. and McGiff, J.C. (1981). Metabolism of prostacyclin: formation of an active metabolites in the liver. *Federation Proceedings,* **40,** 2001 – 2004
185. Brash, A.R., Jackson, E.K., Saggese, C.A., Lawson, J.A., Oates, J.A. and Fitzgerald, G.A. (1983). Metabolic disposition of prostacyclin in humans.*Journal of Pharmacology and Experimental Therapeutics,***226,** 78 – 87
186. Hagen A.A., White, R.P. and Robertson, J.T., (1979). Synthesis of prostaglandins and thromboxane B_2 by cerebral arteries. *Stroke,***10,** 306 – 309
187. Gaudet, R.J., Maurer, P., Levine, L. and Moskowitz, M.A. (1979). Prostoglandins: accumulation in brain after transient ischemia and in vitro synthesis by cerebral microvessels. *Headache,* **19,** 245
188. Wolfe, L.S. (1979). Prostacyclin and prostaglandins and their possible role in migraine. *Headache,* **19,** 245
189. Jarman, D.A., Du Boulay, G.H., Kendall, B. and Bouillin, D.J. (1979). Responses of baboon cerebral and extra cerebral activities to prostacyclin and prostaglandin endoperoxide in-vitro and in-vivo. *Journal of Neurology, Neurosurgery and Psychiatry,* **42,** 667 – 686
190. Pickard, J., Tamura, A., Stewart, M., McGeorge, A. and Girch, W. (1980). Prostacyclin, indomethacin and the cerebral circulation. *Brain Research,* **197,** 425 – 431
191. Brown, M.M. and Pickles, H. (1982). Effect of epoprostenol (prostacyclin, PGI_2) on cerebral blood flow in man. *Journal of Neurology, Neurosurgery and Psychiatry,* **45,** 1033 – 1036
192. Peatfield, R.C., Steiner, T.J., Gawel, M.J. and Rose, F.C. (1981). The role of prostacyclinin the pathogenesis of migraine. In Rose, F.C. and Zilkha, K.J. (Eds.). *Progress in Migraine Research, 1.* London: Pitman, 124 – 129
193. Brandt, L., Ljunggren, B., Andersson, K.E., Hindfelt, B. and Uksi, T. (1983). Prostaglan-

din metabolism and prostacyclin in cerebral vasospasm. *General Pharmacology,* **14,** 141–143
194. Hornby, E.J. and Skidmore, I.F. (1982). Evidence that prostaglandin endoperoxides can induce platelet aggregation in the absence of thromboxane A_2 production. *Biochemical Pharmacology,* **31,** 1158–1160
195. Carlson, L.A. Ekelund, L-G. and Oro, L. (1968). Clinical and metabolic effects of different doses of prostaglandin E in man. *Acta Medica Scandinavica,* **183,** 423–430
196. Pickard, J.D., Macdonell, L.A., Mackenzie, E.T. and Harper, A.M. (1977). Prostaglandin-induced effects in the primate cerebral circulation. *European Journal of Phamacology,* **43,**343–351
197. Williams, T.J. (1979). Prostaglandin E_2, prostaglandin I_2 and the vascular changes of inflammation. *British Journal of Pharmacology,* **65,** 517–524
198. Gorman, R.R. (1979). Modulation of human platelet function by prostacyclin and thromboxane A_2. *Federation Proceedings,* **38,**83–88
199. Parantainen, J. and Vapaatalo, H. (1983). Prostaglandins and migraine. *Trends in Pharmacological Science,* **4,** 379–381
200. Anthony, M. (1976). Plasma free fatty acids and prostaglandin E_1 in migraine andstress. *Headache,* **16,** 58–63
201. Amroyan E.A. (1981). *In Prostaglandins and Thromboxanes* (Ed. Forster, W.). Jena: Fischer Verlag, 157–158. Cited by Parantainen and Vapaatalo (199)
202. Vardi, J., Flecher, S., Alguati, A.,Regev, I. and Ayalon, D. (1983). Prostaglandin E_2 levels in the saliva of common migrainous women. *Headache,* **23,**59–61
203. Peatfield, R.C., Gawel, M.J. and Rose, F.C. (1981). The effect of infused prostacyclin in migraine and cluster headache. *Headache,* **21,** 190–196
204. Raichle, M.E. (1983). The pathophysiology of brain ischemia. *Annals of Neurology,* **13,** 2–10

4

Biochemical changes probably related to the precipitation of migraine

A number of the biochemical abnormalities reported in migraine sufferers appear related to mechanisms which precipitate attacks and thus set in train the biochemical changes (such as those considered in the previous chapter) which actually produce the manifestations of migraine. Those described biochemical changes which appear to play a precipitating role in migraine involve alterations in circulating (a) glucose;(b) free fatty acids;(c) tyramine, phenylethylamine and their conjugating enzyme phenylsulphotransferase;(d) sex and hypothalamic hormones;(e) complement and immunoglobulins and;(f) an as yet unidentified platelet-active factor.

4.1 GLUCOSE

The clinical observation that fasting sometimes precipitates migraine attacks inevitably gave rise to the suggestion that hypoglycaemia might activate the disorder.

4.1.1 Biology

Glucose, via glucose-6-phosphate, is a major source of cellular energy and, in neural tissue, is virtually the only source of energy. Cells take up glucose from the blood by virtue of a membrane transport process facilitated by insulin. The hexose subsequently forms a 6-phosphate ester which then either undergoes anaerobic glycolysis or is polymerised into glycogen, an intracellular energy store. Plasma glucose levels are maintained by the interplay of glucose entry into the blood stream (from its sites of absorption from the alimentary tract and sites of gluconeogenesis) and glucose exit from the blood stream (due to glucose movement into cells under the influence of insulin, and rarely due to renal loss of glucose if renal tubular cell resorptive capacity is outstripped).

Physiological values for fasting plasma glucose concentration are in the range 70–115 mg/100ml.

4.1.2 Glucose changes in migraine

Blau and Cumings[1], redescribed in part by Blau *et al.*[2], subjected 12 migraine sufferers to a 7-hour overnight fast. Next morning six subjects developed migraine before eating, and another two experienced the disorder following breakfast. However no subject had hypoglycaemia on measurement of blood glucose concentration. Blau and Pyke[3] investigated the relation between the onset of diabetes mellitus and migraine and noted a tendency for migraine to lessen after diabetes developed. In four of their diabetic subjects nocturnal hypoglycaemia precipitated migraine attacks. Pearce[4] found insulin-induced hypoglycaemia precipitated headache in two out of 20 migraineurs but in no matched control subjects. Hockaday *et al.*[5] studied ten persons known to develop migraine in relation to hunger. After a 10 hour fast these subjects were given a 50 g glucose load. Half the subjects experienced headache, but there was no fall in blood glucose levels before the headache began. Two years later Hockaday *et al.*[6] gave intravenous glucose and intravenous saline on separate occasions to nine migraineurs known for their tendency to develop attacks when hungry. Six out of the nine experienced migraine when given glucose, but only two of the nine when given saline. After the intravenous glucose administration, blood glucose levels fell more slowly in the migraineurs than in controls. Further, fasting plasma lactate levels tended to be lower in the migraineurs. These findings were interpreted as suggesting that there was decreased cellular uptake of glucose in the migraineurs, possibly due to a degree of insulin resistance. Shaw *et al.*[7] tended to corroborate this result when they found impairment of glucose tolerance in glucose tolerance tests carried out after an overnight fast during as compared with between, migraine attacks in six subjects. However these workers considered that the decreased glucose tolerance was due to the presence of increased free fatty acids and ketones. Plasma insulin levels decreased during the migraine. McLoughlin *et al.*[8] also noted decreased plasma insulin levels during migraine attacks. It should be pointed out that Nader *et al.*[9] had earlier failed to produce migraine by using the same manoeuvres that were successful in the hands of Hockaday *et al.*[6] and which led to the conclusions stated immediately above. In the hours prior to the onset of headache in a group of migraine sufferers, Hsu *et al.*[10] found no change in blood glucose (or insulin) levels. Dexter *et al.*[11] found changes consistent with a degree of reactive hypoglycaemia in 56 out of 74 migraineurs, but they studied no control group. They claimed that a six meal-a-day high-protein diet improved the migraine in 75% of their cases.

There do not seem to have been subsequent published investigations on blood (or plasma) glucose in migraine.

4.1.3 Interpretation of circulating glucose changes in migraine

Even in that group of migraineurs whose attacks are fairly consistently induced by hunger, there is little laboratory evidence that hypoglycaemia produces the attacks. This of course does not necessarily mean that hypoglycaemia is incapable of producing migraine. Blau and Pyke[3] did note hypoglycaemia-associated migraine in a few diabetics. Further evidence as to this possibility is awaited. The available experimental data simply mean that if fasting activates migraine it usually does so by some means other than by causing hypoglycaemia. It should be noted that hypoglycaemia may cause a 3 or 4 fold increase in circulating noradrenaline levels, but a 50 fold increase in circulating adrenaline concentrations[12]. Thus hypoglycaemia could activate migraine via the catecholaminergic mechanisms discussed in Section 3.2.3.

The observation of Hockaday *et al.*[6] and Shaw *et al.*[7] that glucose handling was altered in certain migraneurs in an experimental situation requires confirmation in spontaneous attacks of migraine. It also requires further investigations as to mechanism, before it can be interpreted and set in perspective in relation to any concept of the biochemical events of migraine. It is quite possible that any abnormality found in this circumstance may represent a consequence of migraine, rather than a cause.

4.2 CIRCULATING FREE FATTY ACIDS

The clinical observation that, in some migraine sufferers, attacks are precipitated by intake of various dairy foods (such as cheese or cream) raised the possibility that altered lipid metabolism may play a role in activating the migraine mechanism.

4.2.1 Biology

Lipid biochemistry is complex and the subject of an extensive literature. However, excluding the eicosanoids (see Section 3.6.), the only lipids so far studied in migraine appear to be the free fatty acids.

The free (that is, unesterified) fatty acids are present in circulating blood as the result of several processes:(a) absorption from the alimentary tract; (b) hydrolysis of various fatty acid esters;and (c) entry from cells after intracellular synthesis (ultimately from glucose). Certain (essential) fatty acids, with double bonds at carbon atoms further from the carboxylate tail than C_9 (such as linoleic acid), cannot be synthesised in animals and must be provided by the diet. Only 3–10% of the total fatty acid in serum is unesterified: the remaining fatty acid is in the form of glycerol, phosphoric acid or cholesterol esters; the free fatty acids bond reversibly to plasma albumin. In serum from normal adults the free fatty acid level is in the range 100–350 mg/l. The major acids are palmitic (28%), stearic (15%), linoleic (13%) and oleic (26%). Their formulae are shown in Figure 4.1.

$CH_3(CH_2)_{14}.COOH$ –palmitic acid

$CH_3(CH_2)_{16}.COOH$ –stearic acid

$CH_3(CH_2)_7.CH{=}CH.(CH_2)_2.COOH$ –oleic acid

$CH_3(CH_2)_4.CH{=}CH.CH_2.CH{=}CH.(CH_2)_7COOH$ –linoleic acid

$CH_3(CH_2)_4.CH{=}CH.CH_2.CH{=}CH.CH_2.CH{=}CH.CH_2.CH{=}CH(CH_2)_3.COOH$

–arachidonic acid

Figure 4.1 Formulae for free (unesterified) fatty acids

Linoleic acid is a precursor of arachidonic acid, the progenitor of the eicosanoids.

4.2.2 Free fatty acid changes in migraine

In their studies in fasted migraineurs described in Section 4.1.2. Hockaday *et al.*[5] noted a rise in circulating free fatty acid levels prior to the onset of headache. There was a further elevation in free fatty acid level during the headache phase (despite the giving of a 50 g glucose load). In the subsequent study of Hockaday *et al.*[6], again in migraineurs prone to develop attacks when fasted, an almost completely contrary finding was obtained. Attacks were induced by intravenous glucose administration and tended to occur at the time of lowest circulating free fatty acid levels. Further, plasma free fatty acid levels tended to fall more in the migraineurs than in control subjects after the glucose load. Shaw *et al.*[7] noted increased circulating free fatty acid levels, paralleling increased blood glycerol levels, during migraine attacks in six subjects who had intravenous glucose tolerance tests carried out following an overnight fast.

The matter was reinvestigated by Hsu *et al.*[10]. These workers followed the levels of a number of circulating endogenous biological substances before and during migraine attacks. Despite the biogenic amine alterations alluded to earlier (Section 3.2), there was no change in free fatty acid, glucose or circulating insulin levels in the pre-headache phase. It may be worth mentioning that Hsu *et al.*[10] had infused small amounts of heparin to keep a venous cannula patent during their studies. Possibly the heparin altered fatty acid levels. By way of contrast to Hsu *et al.*[10], in the same year Anthony[13] expanded on his earlier[14] publication and described elevated free fatty acid levels in platelet-poor plasma in eight out of ten migraine attacks studied. The mean increase in fatty acid level was 46%, the increases in levels of palmitic, stearic, oleic and linoleic acid being, respectively, 36, 80, 95 and 137.5%. Anthony[15] appears to have described this study again, in relation to his investigation of altered sympathetic activity in migraine. However the later report included the additional information that stearic and palmitic acid levels had increased in nine out of ten attacks, and linoleic acid in all 10 attacks.

Thus the findings in migraine in relation to circulating free fatty acids show inconsistencies between the various investigations. Assuming that the measurements were accurate in the first place, it appears that free fatty acid levels may or may not be raised prior to the onset of migraine headache, and, perhaps more consistently, may rise during attacks.

4.2.3 Interpretation of free fatty acid changes in migraine

4.2.3.1 Relation to the production of migraine

Assuming that circulating free fatty acid levels do rise in migraine, and since linoleic acid is a precursor of the eicosanoids (see Section 4.2.1),one may speculate that increased free fatty acid levels in migraine could lead to increased availability of various vasoactive eicosanoids. However, the relevant eicosanoids have transient existences, and appear to be derived entirely from membrane lipids. Therefore it appears unlikely that increased free fatty acid availability would exert a significant driving effect on eicosanoid production. An alternative, and perhaps more likely possibility, is that the increased fatty acids may activate platelets to cause serotonin release[13]. This, in turn, might activate other platelets. All the four fatty acids studied by Anthony[13,15] are capable of activating platelets. Seen in this light, the fatty acid changes could initiate, and maintain, the platelet and serotonin mechanisms which provide a reasonably plausible, though incomplete, explanation for the biochemical pathogenesis of migraine.

4.2.3.2 Cause of free fatty acid level alterations

Dairy food intake, with resultant raised plasma free (and esterified) fatty acid levels, could explain migraine activation in individuals whose attacks follow such food intake. However it should be pointed out that raised fatty acid levels do not appear to have been demonstrated in these circumstances in migraineurs.

It is known that altered sympathetic nervous system activity, and raised plasma noradrenaline levels, can be associated with the appearance of increased circulating free fatty acid concentrations. Serotonin infusion causes raised plasma free fatty acid levels[14]. Evidence of raised plasma noradrenaline levels prior to the onset of, and during migraine, is described in Section 3.2. Anthony[15] has brought together several lines of biochemical evidence in arguing that there is increased sympathetic activity during migraine attacks and this explains the circulating fatty acid and the catecholamine changes of this disorder. In a general way, it is not difficult to accept that the pain and distress of migraine might activate the sympathetic nervous system.

Thus there seems a reasonably adequate explanation for an elevation of circulating free fatty acid levels in migraine, should such an elevation occur, and there is a plausible basis for these fatty acids playing a causative role in the disorder, via platelet activation. The main uncertainty lies in whether, and if so at what stage of the evolution of attacks, the reported fatty acid changes really do occur.

4.3 TYRAMINE, PHENYLETHYLAMINE AND PHENOLSULPHOTRANSFERASE

Another aspect of the possible relation between food factors and migraine provocation has been investigated chemically. Chocolate, cheese and citrus fruits, all with appreciable amine contents, are among the more common precipitants of attacks in those with so-called 'dietary' migraine. Therefore the role of certain amines in producing migraine is worth examination. The subject has been reviewed by Glover *et al.*[16].

4.3.1 Biology

4.3.1.1 Tyramine

Tyramine is the decarboxylation product of the aminoacid tyrosine. A series of phenolic amines, analogous to the catecholamines, can be derived from tyrosine (see Section 3.2.1.1) (Figure 4.2).

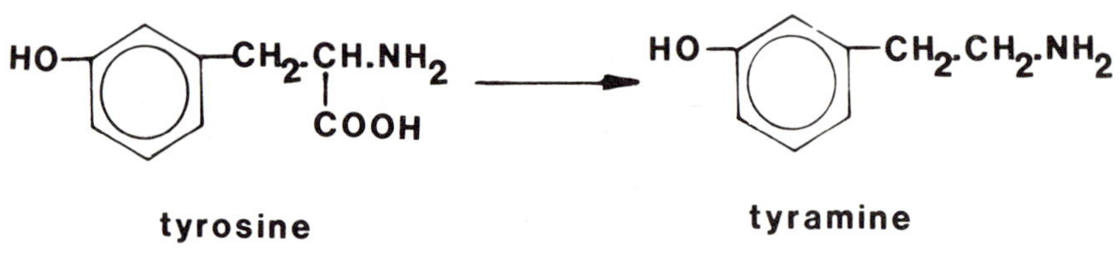

Figure 4.2 Formation of tyramine

The decarboxylation can occur in various animal tissues, including the central nervous system, and in bacteria. Tyramine in the body may be of dietary origin (from, for instance, chocolate) or it may possibly be formed in the gut lumen from bacterial decomposition of tyrosine and then be absorbed. It may also be formed within the body from metabolism of tyrosine. Tyramine is oxidatively deaminated by monoamine oxidase (both type A and type B). Since there is a substantial amount of type A monoamine oxidase in the intestinal wall it might be expected that, in normal circumstances, an appreciable portion of an oral tyramine load would be deaminated before it could gain access to the circulation.

circulation.

4.3.1.2 Phenylethylamine

Phenylethylamine is the decarboxylation product of phenylalanine, and is formed in tissues, including catecholaminergic neurons[17], as result of metabolism of the aminoacid. Its mechanism of formation is analogous to that of tyramine. Phenylethylamine is a substrate for monoamine oxidase type B, but not type A. Hence, unlike tyramine, phenylethylamine of dietary origin (there are appreciable amounts in chocolate) would be unlikely to undergo metabolic inactivation during its absorption through the gut wall into the circulation. Unlike many amines, phenylethylamine will cross the blood – brain barrier[17,18].

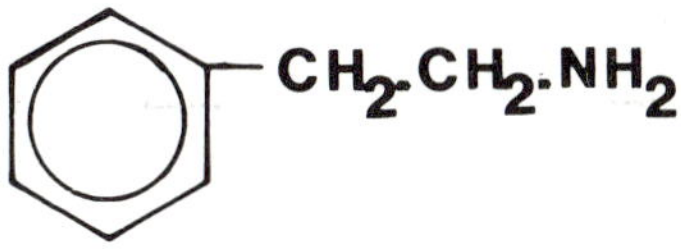

phenylethylamine

McCulloch and Harper[19-21] studied the effect of intracarotid administration of phenylethylamine on cerebral blood flow in anaesthesised baboons. At low concentration the amine increased cerebral blood flow and O_2 consumption. At doses some 50 times greater it reduced the blood flow and oxygen consumption. McCullough and Harper stated that phenylethylamine caused the release of noradrenaline.

4.3.1.3 Phenolsulphotransferase

Until recently, comparatively little attention has been paid to this enzyme. It catalyses the formation of sulphate conjugates of a number of phenolic compounds, and this, for practical purposes, inactivates them (Figure 4.3).

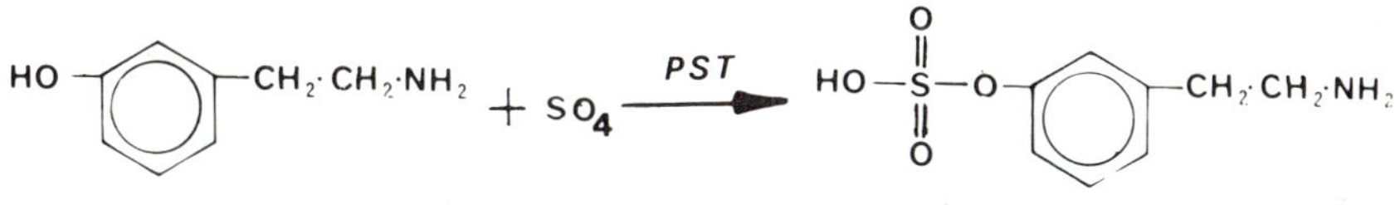

tyramine **tyramine sulphate**

Figure 4.3 The sulphation of tyrosine

Phenolsulphotransferase occurs in platelets, in the jejunum, adrenal and brain. The enzyme appears to exist in two forms, the M (monoamine) and P (phenol) types[22]. The M form catalyses the sulphation of a number of phenolic amines and catecholamines, but not phenylethylamine[16]. The P form has no known endogenous substrate, but catalyses the sulphate conjugation of phenol itself, and of salicylamide.

4.3.2 Changes in the amines, and in phenolsulphotranferase, in migraine

Hanington *et al.*[23] fed oral tyramine to 45 dietary migraineurs, and to a larger control group, and noted a significantly increased production of headaches in the dietary migraine group. Youdim *et al.*[35] stated that tyramine provoked attacks in 30% of cases of classical migraine. In contrast Moffett *et al.*[(24)] and Ryan[25] failed to confirm this finding in dietary migraineurs. Shaw *et al.*[26] also failed to activate migraine in this way. However, they gave the tyramine with parnate, a monoamine oxidase inhibitor. This confounded interpretation of the finding as the metabolism of various endogenous amines would probably also have been altered. Ziegler and Stewart[27] studied a population of 80 migraineurs whose attacks were not necessarily of dietary origin. These workers carried out a double-blind study of the effects of 200 mg tyramine and placebo, and found no increased tendency of tyramine to induce migraine attacks. Ziegler *et al.*[28] had earlier shown that oral tyramine intake in 26 fasted migraineurs did not alter whole blood serotonin content. Ghose et al.[29] reported that intravenously administered tyramine was more likely to induce migraine in sufferers from the disorder than in control subjects. Peatfield *et al.*[30] obtained a similar result. Of course, in the latter two studies, the route of tyramine administration bypassed the alimentary tract wall, with its monoamine oxidase activity capable of degrading tyramine. Kohlenberg[31] critically reviewed published work on the role of tyramine in migraine production. He concluded that the amine precipitated attacks in some 5% of migraineurs.

So far as we have been able to trace, there has been no measurement of plasma amine concentration changes (if any) produced by tyramine administration. The available data do not permit any reasonably based conclusion that tyramine plays a role in spontaneous or dietary migraine.

Sandler *et al.*[32] on the basis of a report that phenylethylamine was present at significant concentrations in chocolate, gave this amine by mouth to 36 persons with reputed chocolate-induced migraine in a placebo-controlled study. Phenylethylamine appeared capable of inducing migraine attacks in half these persons, after a delay of some 12 hours. Sandler *et al.*[32] noted a decreased capacity of migraineurs' platelets to oxidise phenylethylamine, probably a consequence of reduce monoamine oxidase activity (see Section 3.3.1).

Smith *et al.*[33] reported that dietary migraineurs excreted less free and conjugated tyramine in urine after an oral tyramine load than did control subjects. However, in a subsequent study[34] these same workers appear to have arrived at a contrary conclusion as regards urinary tyramine (which was present only as conjugates). Youdim *et al.*[35] found that, after a dietary load of tyramine, migraineurs excreted more of the amine in urine in a non-conjugated form than did normal persons. They suspected there was a defect in sulphate conjugation in migraineurs. Smith *et al.*[36] arrived at a similar conclusion, based on their own study, following Mullen and Smith's[37] demonstration that the conjugate excreted in decreased amount in dietary migraine was tyramine-*O*-

sulphate. Littlewood *et al.*[38] studied platelet phenolsulphotransferase activity in 19 dietary migraineurs, 26 control migraineurs and 17 non-migrainous control subjects. Platelet levels of the P type of phenolsulphotransferse activity were substantially reduced in the dietary migraineurs, while levels of the M type of enzyme were reduced to an extent that reached the borderline of statistical significance.

4.3.3 Interpretation of amine and phenolsulphotransferase changes in migraine

The evidence incriminating tyramine in the pathogenesis of dietary migraine is far from unequivocal, and that incriminating phenylethylamine depends on a single study which has not yet been repeated. The work on altered platelet phenolsulphotransferase activity in migraine comes from a single group of investigators who, in the same study, obtained values for platelet monoamine oxidase activity different from those found in all their previous work. The type of phenolsulphotransferase that was most affected was one for which there is no known endogenous substrate. One should acknowledge the possibility that, if phenolsulphotransferase is similarly deficient in the intestinal wall, some as yet unrecognised dietary phenolic compound could reach the circulation in increased quantities and there activate the migraine mechanism. However such a proposal is in large measure speculation. The possibility canvassed may be correct, but further work must be done before it can provide a reasonable basis for any adequate hypothesis of migraine pathogenesis.

4.4 SEX HORMONES

There is a generally recognised relation between menstruation and migraine in females. Such an association occurred in 24 out of 138 women in the series of Epstein *et al.*[39]. Green[40] traced a report of this relation dating from as early as 1764 and the association was commented on by Latham, in 1872[41]. Intake of oral contraceptives with a higher oestrogen content than at present often precipitated migraine[42,43]. Contemporary combination oral contraceptives still tend to increase the number of migraine attacks in women[44]. According to Hanington *et al.*[45] 25% of women at a migraine clinic had attacks associated with oral contraceptive intake. The attacks had decreased in all within 4–6 months of stopping the Pill. Whitty *et al.*[46] suggested that withdrawal of added progesterone precipitates migraine related to oral contraceptives. Migraine often eases or disappears during pregnancy. These well-attested facts inevitably point to the question of the relation between hormones mediating sexual function in females and the production of migraine. Unfortunately there is relatively little precise information available about this matter.

Epstein *et al.*[39] found no specific changes in various sex hormone levels associated with the advent of menstrual migraine. Nader *et al.*[9] noted that a number of factors which seem related to the development of migraine, e.g. oestrogens, serotonin, exercise and stress, produced raised prolactin levels. To assess the role of prolactin in migraine they attempted to induce attacks of the disorder by fasting subjects, and then giving them intravenous glucose. Even when prolactin levels were also raised by giving chlorpromazine simultaneously, no headaches resulted. Further, alcohol, which can produce migraine in some subjects, did not alter plasma prolactin levels in these subjects. On the basis of these considerations and their rather complicated experimental design, these authors concluded that there was no evidence that prolactin was involved in the production of migraine. Subsequently Wainscott[47] failed to find any alterations in plasma prolactin levels prior to migraine attacks, and Polleri *et al.*[48,49] reported that the time courses of plasma prolactin levels over 24 hours did not differ between migraineurs and controls.

Nattero[50] and Nattero *et al.*[51] reported a study in which women with regular premenstrual migraine attacks on the 26th day of their menstrual cycle were found to have plasma oestrogen and progesterone levels almost double those of controls. Prolactin concentrations also were increased at this time though not to a statistically significant extent.

Somerville[52-54] carried out a systematic investigation of the role of female sex hormones in a group of five women with menstrual migraine and in a control group of five normal women. The onset of the migraine occurred during or at the end of the phase of falling plasma progesterone levels. There was no statistically significant difference between progesterone levels in the migraineurs and the control subjects. When Somerville injected progesterone daily to prevent the premenstrual fall in plasma progesterone levels the menses were delayed, but the migraine still tended to occur at its usual time. It therefore appeared that progesterone was not causally related to the migraine. However the spontaneous migraine in these women also occurred at a time of falling plasma oestrogen levels. Injecting oestrogens in the latter phase of the menstrual cycle in these menstrual migraineurs did not alter their plasma progesterone levels, and did not delay the onset of the menses, but did postpone by several days the onset of migraine. Thus it appeared that a fall in plasma oestrogen levels would precipitate migraine, at least in menstrual migraineurs. This conclusion was corroborated by the observation of Dennerstein *et al.*[55] that, in females who had undergone a surgically-induced menopause, withdrawal of oestrogen therapy was associated with an increase in headache. Chaudhuri[56] noted that oestrogen therapy decreased the severity of migraine in two women with premature ovarian failure.

Although the body of evidence regarding circulating ostrogens and migraine is not large, it does appear internally consistent and fits with clinical experience. In at least some women who tend to get migraine premenstrually, falling plasma oestrogen levels seem to be associated with the development of migraine attacks. How the fall in oestrogen levels can activate the migraine mechanism remains unclear. One might speculate that the oestrogens alter platelet function, but evidence as to a more detailed mechanism of action is as yet wanting. The association between oestrogen changes and migraine is probably limited to a relatively selected group of migraineurs , and is not a general mechanism in the disorder. Thus Horthe *et al.*[57] found no differences in plasma oestrogen levels between a group of female migraineurs (who were not specifically mentioned to be menstrual migraineurs) and control subjects, though there were higher progesterone levels in the last 3 days of the menstrual cycle in the migraineurs. At the times of 8 migraine attacks there was no abrupt alteration in plasma levels of the female sex hormones.

4.5 COMPLEMENT AND IMMUNOGLOBULINS

Lord and Duckworth[58] reported changes in immunoglobulins and in complement in migraine. They found increased levels of IgA in cases of prodromal migraine, increased levels of IgA and IgG in cases of common migraine and increased levels of IgA, IgG and IgM in non-prodromal migraineurs who developed neurological deficits during the headache phase of their episodes. There was evidence of complement activation during the migraine attacks: levels of C_4 and C_5 were decreased, and also levels of C_4, C_{1S} and $C_{1(1)}$ early in the attacks. Complement break-down products were present 3 hours before the headaches began, and complement seemed to return to normal by a late stage of the attacks. It was suggested that there might be a late-stage, short-duration, immune reaction during migraine.

Subsequently Lord and Duckworth[59] contradicted their previous finding and indicated that serum complement was not altered during prodromal migraine, but only in non-prodromal migraine. Further, Moore *et al.*[60] described a careful study in which they found no difference in immunoglobulin, complement or immune complex levels in 30 migraineurs, as compared with controls. They also found no differences between sufferers from common and classical migraine in respect to these parameters. Behan *et al.*[61] also failed to find any evidence of complement activation during migraine attacks and Sovak *et al.*[62] detected no difference in C_1 inhibitor levels between migraineurs and normal control subjects. More recently Jerzmanowski and Klimek[63] studied 54 migraineurs and noted reduced levels of C_3 and IgA, but normal levels of C_4, total complement, IgG and IgM. They interpreted these findings as suggesting activation of the alternative pathway of the complement system.

When there is disagreement to this extent between the various groups who have studied these matters it is difficult to know where the truth lies. The validity of the observation that complement break-down products are present prior to migraine attacks must be suspect. The postulated immune reaction leading to complement breakdown could be a possible aetiological factor in migraine. Since this possibility cannot yet be discarded, the mechanisms which might be involved are discussed below.

The complement system is a set of some 18 protein moieties which may interact serially after initial activation. Factors which trigger the complement system include contact with antigen – antibody complexes or activated factor XII. Triggering the complement system sets in train a sequence of reactions in which activation of one stage causes the activated molecule to exert an endopeptidase effect on the next component of the complement system and this component, in turn, on a further component, or components, and so on. Finally a cell membrane damaging complex is formed. Thus the presence of complement breakdown products can serve as an indication that an antigen – antibody reaction has occurred. However activated factor XII can also cause complement breakdown, and factor XII activation is also a precursor for kinin formation (see Section 3.5). It is not yet unequivocally proven that kinin formation does occur in migraine, but if it did, and if complement breakdown products do occur in plasma in migraine, one might consider the possibility that activation of factor XII was the common basis for both changes. It would then appear worth seeking causes of activation of factor XII in trying to understand the mechanisms of migraine. However, this whole area, as yet, lacks a well-founded basis of experimental observation. Therefore the suggestions offered above should be treated with considerable caution.

It is known that aggregated circulating IgG_1, IgG_2, IgG_3 and IgG_4 and normal IgG complexes can all cause platelets to aggregate and release serotonin[64]. If there really are IgG changes in migraine, these may represent a mechanism whereby the attacks develop.

4.6 THE UNIDENTIFIED CIRCULATING FACTOR WHICH ALTERS PLATELET FUNCTION

Several groups of workers have detected the presence in plasma during migraine attacks of a factor which appears to activate platelets and promotes their aggregation (see Section 3.1.2.1). The chemical nature of this factor (or factors) is as yet unknown.

Anthony *et al.*[65] described studies in which they incubated platelets from migraineurs when headache-free with platelet-poor plasma from the same subjects obtained during attacks of migraine. The plasma collected during attacks appeared to contain a factor which caused serotonin loss from the platelets. This factor could pass through a filter with a molecular weight cut off of 50 000 daltons. This report appears to have been the first observation of such a circulating serotonin-releasing factor in migraine. Subsequently Dvilansky *et al.*[66] and Mück-Seler *et al.*[67,68] published data generally supporting Anthony's finding. Mück-Seler *et al.*[67,68] showed that (i) platelet serotonin content fell by a mean of 22% when platelets from headache-free migraineurs were incubated with platelet-poor plasma collected during a migraine attack (ii) platelet serotonin content did not fall when platelets from headache-free migraineurs were incubated with platelet-poor plasma from persons who did not suffer from migraine, and (iii) platelet serotonin content did not fall when platelets from non-migraineurs were incubated with platelet-poor plasma from migraineurs collected during migraine attacks. It thus appeared that there was both an abnormality of the platelets of migraineurs, and that during migraine attacks a substance appeared in plasma which promoted serotonin release from these abnormal platelets. Launay *et al.*[69] detected the presence in plasma during migraine attacks of a factor which interfered with platelet uptake of serotonin.

Anthony[15] suggested that the serotonin-releasing factor may be one or other of the free fatty acids whose plasma levels rise during migraine (see Section 4.2). However no studies appear to have been published describing systematic attempts to determine the chemical nature of the serotonin-releasing factor. There may, of course, be more than one such factor, but this appears to be a very promising area to investigate in any search for the biochemical basis of migraine. Bruyn's[70] suggestion that the factor is a neuropeptide comprising 130–140 aminoacid residues which is released from the hypothalamus, may prove valid. The known platelet-activating factor[71] is another possibility. It is of low molecular weight, is released from platelets and macrophages, and appears to aggregate platelets by reactions that do not involve eicosanoid mechanisms.

References

1. Blau, J.N. and Cumings, J.N. (1966). Method of precipitating and preventing some migraine attacks. *British Medical Journal,* **2,** 1242–1243
2. Blau, J.N., Horsfield, D., Quick, J and Cumings, J.N. (1967). The production of migraine and biochemical changes in induced attacks. In Smith, R. (ed.). *Background to Migraine.* London: Heinemann, 146–153
3. Blau, J.N. and Pyke, D.A. (1970). Effect of diabetes on migraine. *Lancet,* **2,** 241–243
4. Pearce, J. (1971). Insulin induced hypoglycaemia in migraine. *Journal of Neurology, Neurosurgery and Psychiatry,* **34,** 154–156
5. Hockaday, J.W., Williamson, D.H. and Whitty, C.W.M. (1971). Blood glucose levels and fatty acid metabolism in migraine related to fasting. *Lancet,* **1,** 1153–1156
6. Hockaday, J.M., Williamson, D.H. and Alberti, K.G.M.M. (1973). Effects of intravenous glucose on some blood metabolites and hormones in migraine subjects. In Cumings, J.N. (ed.) *Background to Migraine.* London: Heinemann. 99–111
7. Shaw, S.W.J., Johnson, R.W. and Keogh, H.J. (1977). Metabolic changes during glucose tolerance tests in migraine attacks. *Journal of the Neurological Sciences,* **33,** 51–59
8. McLoughlin, J.C., Buchanan, K.D. and Ardill, J.E. (1978). Entero-pancreatic hormones in migraine. *Irish Journal of Medicine,* **147,** 151–155
9. Nader, S., Tulloch, B., Blair, C., Vydelingum, N. and Fraser, T.R. (1974). Is prolactin involved in precipitating migraine? *Lancet,* **2,** 17–19
10. Hsu, L.K.G., Crisp, A.H., Kalucy, R.S., Koval, J., Chen, C.N., Carruthers, M. and Zilkha, K.J. (1978). Nocturnal plasma levels of catecholamines, tryptophan, glucose, and free fatty acids and the sleeping electroencephalographs of subjects experiencing early morning migraine. In Greene, R. (ed.). *Current Concepts in Migraine Research.* New York: Raven Press, 121–130
11. Dexter, J.D., Roberts, J. and Byer, J.A. (1978). The five hour glucose tolerance test and effect of low sucrose diet in migraine. *Headache,* **18,** 91–94
12. Bravo, E.L. and Tazari, R.C. (1982). Plasma catecholamines in clinical investigation: a useful index or a meaningless number. *Journal of Laboratory and Clinical Medicine,* **100,** 155–160
13. Anthony, M. (1978). Role of individual free fatty acids in migraine. *Research and Clinical Studies in Headache,* **6,** 110–116
14. Anthony, M. (1976). Plasma free fatty acids and prostaglandin E_1 in migraine and stress. *Headache,* **16,** 58–63
15. Anthony, M. (1981). Biochemical indices of sympathetic activity in migraine. *Cephalalgia,* **1,** 83–89
16. Glover, V., Littlewood, J., Sandler, M., Peatfield, R., Petty, R. and Rose, F.C. (1983). Biochemical predisposition to dietary migraine: the role of phenolsulphotransferase. *Headache,* **23,** 53–58
17. Sabelli, H.C., Borison, R.L., Diamond, B.I., Havdala, H.S. and Narasimhachari, N. (1918). Phenylethylamine and brain function. *Biochemical Pharmacology,* **27,** 1707–1711
18. Oldendorf, W.H. (1971). Brain uptake of radiolabelled amino acids, amines and hexoses after arterial injection. *American Journal of Physiology,* **221,** 1629–1639
19. McCulloch, J. and Harper, A.M. (1977). Phenylethylamine, migraine and the cerebral circulations. *Acta Neurologica Scandinavica,* Suppl. **56,** 202–203
20. McCulloch, J. and Harper, A.M. (1977). Phenylethylamine and cerebral blood flow. *Neurology,* **27,** 817–821
21. McCulloch, J. and Harper, A.M. (1978). Phenylethylamine and cerebral circula-

tion, In Greene, R. (ed.) *Current Concepts in Migraine Research.* New York: Raven Press, 85–88

22. Rein, G., Glover, V. and Sandler, M. (1982). Multiple forms of sulphotransferase in human tissues: selective inhibition by dichloronitrophenol. *Biochemical Pharmacology,* **31,** 1893–1897
23. Hanington, E., Horn, M. and Wilkinson, M. (1970). Further observations on the effects of tyramine. In Cochrane, A.L. (ed.) *Background to Migraine.* London: Heinemann, 113– 119
24. Moffett, A., Swash, M. and Scott, D.F. (1972). Effect of tyramine in migraine: a double-blind study. *Journal of Neurology, Neurosurgery and Psychiatry,* **35,** 496–499
25. Ryan, R.E. Jr. (1974). A clinical study of tyramine as an etiological factor in migraine. *Headache,* **14,** 43–48
26. Shaw, S.W.J., Johnson, R.W. and Keogh, H.J. (1978). Oral tyramine in dietary migraine sufferers. In Greene, R. (ed.) *Current Concepts in Migraine Research.* New York: Raven Press, 31–39
27. Ziegler, D.K. and Stewart, R. (1977). Failure of tyramine to induce migraine. *Neurology,* **27,** 725–726
28. Ziegler, D.K., Hassanein, R.S. and Ward, D.F. (1976). Migraine, tyramine and blood serotonin. *Headache,* **16,** 53– 57
29. Ghose, K., Coppen, A. and Carroll, D. (1977). Intravenous tyramine response in migraine before and during treatment with indoramin. *British Medical Journal,* **1,** 1191–1193
30. Peatfield, R., Littlewood, J.T., Sandler, M. and Rose, F.C. (1983). Pressor sensitivity to tyramine in patients with headache: relationship to platelet monoamine oxidase and to dietary provocation. *Journal of Neurology, Neurosurgery and Psychiatry,* **46,** 827–831
31. Kohlenberg, R.J. (1982). Tyramine sensitivity in dietary migraine: a critical review. *Headache,* **22,** 30–34
32. Sandler, M., Youdim, M.B.H. and Hanington, E. (1974). A phenylethylamine oxidising defect in migraine. *Nature,* **250,** 335–337
33. Smith, I., Kellow, A.H. and Hanington, E. (1970). Tyramine metabolism in dietary migraine. In Cochrane, A.L. (ed.) *Background to Migraine.* London: Heinemann, 120–124
34. Smith, I., Gordon, A.J., Hanington, E., Marsh, S.E. and Wilkinson, M.I.P. (1973). Studies of tyramine metabolism in migraine patients and control subjects. In Cumings, J.N. (ed.) *Background to Migraine.* London: Heinemann. 34– 39
35. Youdim, M.B.H., Bonham-Carter, S., Sandler, M., Hanington, E. and Wilkinson, M. (1977). Conjugation defect in tyramine- sensitive migraine. *Nature,* **230,** 127–128
36. Smith, I., Kellow, J.H., Mullen, P.E. and Hanington, E. (1971). Dietary migraine and tyramine metabolism. *Nature.* **230,** 246–248
37. Mullen, P.E. and Smith, I. (1971). Tyramine metabolism and migraine: a metabolic defect. *British Journal of Pharmacology,* **41,** 413P–414P
38. Littlewood, J., Glover, V., Sandler, M., Petty, R., Peatfield, R. and Rose, F.C. (1982). Platelet phenosulphotransferase deficiency in dietary migraine. *Lancet,* **l,** 983–986
39. Epstein, M.T., Hockaday, J.M. and Hockaday, T.D.R. (1975). Migraine and reproductive hormones throughout the menstrual cycle. *Lancet,* **1,** 543–547
40. Greene, R. (1973). The endocrinology of headache. The Sandoz lecture. In Cumings, J.N. (ed.) *Background to Migraine.* London: Heinemann, 82–92
41. Latham, P.A. (1972). Clinical lectures on nervous or sick headaches. *British Medical Journal,* **1,** 305–306;336– 337
42. Phillips, B.M. (1968). Oral contraceptive drugs and migraine. *British Medical Journal,* **2,** 99
43. Dalton, K. (1976). Migraine and oral contraceptives. *Headache,* **15,** 247–251
44. Ryan, R.E. Snr. (1978). A controlled study of the effect of oral contraceptives on migraine. *Headache,* **17,** 250– 252
45. Hanington, E., Jones, R.L. and Amess, J.A.L. (1982). Platelet aggregation in response to 5-HT in migraine patients taking oral contraceptives. *Lancet,* **1,** 967– 968
46. Whitty, C.W.M., Hockaday, J.M. and Whitty, M.M. (1966). The effects of oral contraceptives on migraine. *Lancet,* **1,** 856–859
47. Wainscott, G. (1978). Prolactin levels during a migraine attack. In Greene, R. (ed.) *Current Concepts in Migraine Research.* New York: Raven Press, 105–109

48. Polleri, A., Nappi, G., Masturzo, P., Martignoni, E., Murialdo, G., Bono, G., Testa, E. and Savoldi, F. (1982). Neuroendocrine approach to headache. *Advances in Neurology,* **33,** 173–182
49. Polleri, A., Nappi, G., Murialdo, G., Bono, G., Martignoni, E. and Savoldi, F. (1982). Changes in the 24-hour prolactin pattern in cluster headache. *Cephalalgia,* **2,** 1–7
50. Nattero, G. (1978). Sex hormones, prolactin levels, osmolality and electrolyte patterns in menstrual migraine – relationship to fluid retention. *Headache,* **18,** 110
51. Nattero, G., Bisbocci, D. and Ceresa, F. (1979). Sex hormones, prolactin levels, osmolarity and electrolyte patterns in menstrual migraine – relationship with fluid retention. *Headache,* **19,** 25–30
52. Somerville, B.W. (1971). The influence of hormonal change upon migraine in women. *Proceedings of the Australian Association of Neurologists* **8,** 47–53
53. Somerville, B.W. (1971). The role of progesterone in menstrual migraine. *Neurology,* **21,** 853–859
54. Somerville, B.W. (1972). The role of estradiol withdrawal in the etiology of menstrual migraine. *Neurology,* **22,** 355– 366
55. Dennerstein, L., Laby, B., Burrows, G.D. and Hyman, G.J. (1978). Headache and sex hormone therapy. *Headache,* **18,** 146–153
56. Chaudhuri, T.K. and Chaudhuri, S.T. (1975). Estrogen therapy for migraine. *Headache,* **15,** 139–141
57. Horthe, C.E., Wainscott, G., Neylan, C. and Wilkinson, M.I.P. (1975). Progesterone, oestradiol and aldosterone levels in plasma during the menstrual cycle of women suffering from migraine. *Journal of Endocrinology,* **65,** 24P
58. Lord, G.D.A. and Duckworth, J.W. (1977). Immunoglobulin and complement studies in migraine. *Headache,* **17,** 163– 168
59. Lord, G.D.A. and Duckworth, J.W. (1978). Complement and immune complex studies in migraine. *Headache,* **18,** 255– 260
60. Moore, T.L., Ryan, R.E. Jr., Pohl, D.A., Roodman, S.T. and Ryan, R.E. Sr. (1980). Immunoglobulin, complement, and immune complex levels during a migraine attack. *Headache,* **20,** 9–12
61. Behan, W.M.H., Behan, P.O. and Durward, W.F. (1981). Complement studies in migraine. *Headache,* **21,** 55–57
62. Sovak, M., Kunzel, M., Dalessio, D.J. and Lang, J.H. (1980). C-1 inhibitor levels in migraineurs and normals. *Headache,* **20,** 132–133
63. Jerzmanowski, A. and Klimek, A. (1983). Immunoglobulins and complement in migraine. *Cephalalgia,* **3,** 119–123
64. Henson, P.M. and Spiegelberg, H.L. (1973). Release of serotonin from human platelets induced by aggregated immunoglobulins of different classes and subclasses. *Journal of Clinical Investigation,* **52,** 1282–1288
65. Anthony, M., Hinterberger, H. and Lance, J.W. (1968). Studies of serotonin metabolism in migraine. *Proceedings of the Australian Association of Neurologists,* **5,** 109– 112
66. Divlansky, A., Rishpon, S., Nathan, I., Zocotow, Z. and Dorczyn, A.D. (1976). Release of platelet 5- hydroxytryptamine by plasma taken from patients during and between migraine attacks. *Pain,* **2,** 315–318
67. Mück-Seler, D., Deanović, Z. and Dupelj, M. (1979). Platelet serotonin (5-HT) and 5-HT releasing factor in plasma of migrainous patients. *Headache,* **19,** 14–17
68. Mück-Seler, D., Deanović, Z. and Dupelj, M. (1982). Serotonin-releasing factors in migrainous patients. *Advances in Neurology,* **33,** 257–264
69. Launay, J.M., Pradalier, A., Dreux, C. and Dry, J. (1982). Platelet serotonin uptake and migraine. *Cephalalgia,* **2,** 57–59
70. Bruyn, G.W. (1982). Cerebral cortex and migraine. In Critchley, M., Friedman, A.P., Gorini, S. and Sicuteri, F. (eds.) Migraine: Physiopathological and Clinical Aspects. *Advances in Neurology,* **33,** 151–169
71. Vargaftig, B.B. and Benveniste, J. (1983). Platelet- activating factor today. *Trends in Pharmacological Sciences,* **4,** 341–343

5

Biochemical changes which appear to be probable consequences of migraine

A number of the biochemical changes reported as occurring in migraine appear to be probable consequences of the various events which are generally accepted as part of migraine. Although in the current state of knowledge these biochemical changes appear to be secondary they should be discussed, not only for completeness but also because, as knowledge grows, they may come to be seen in other than a secondary role.

5.1 GAMMA-AMINOBUTYRATE (GABA)

5.1.1 Biology

γ-Aminobutyrate is an aminoacid whose occurrence in the body is almost entirely confined to neural tissue. The aminoacid serves both as a metabolic intermediate and as a neurotransmitter. It constitutes part of the so-called GABA shunt, which bypasses several steps in the Krebs cycle, as shown in Figure 5.1.

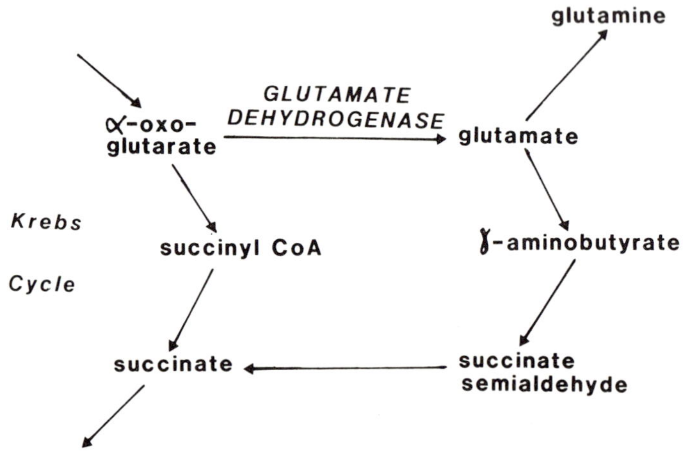

Figure 5.1 The GABA shunt

The stages in the formation and degradation of γ-aminobutyrate are set out in Figure 5.2.

γ-Aminobutyrate serves as an inhibitory neurotransmitter acting at specific receptors of more than one type in the central nervous system. Its action is to cause hyperpolarisation of postsynaptic neuronal cell membranes by increasing their permeability to Cl^-. The action of γ-aminobutyrate, after release from axon terminals, is ended by active reuptake into presynaptic terminals or into glia, or by metabolic degradation, possibly in postsynaptic terminals.

Kelly *et al.*[1] studied the effects of perivascularly administered GABA on cat pial arteries, and showed that concentrations above 10^{-7} mol/l dilate these vessels. This effect is antagonised by picrotoxin or bicuculline, GABA antagonists at receptor sites. These authors point out that the inhibitory effect of GABA on neurotransmission would tend to decrease regional cortical metabolism, and thus, by auto regulation, would diminish regional cerebral blood flow. Therefore the local neuronal effects of increased GABA concentrations, and the direct vascular effects of these, would oppose each other.

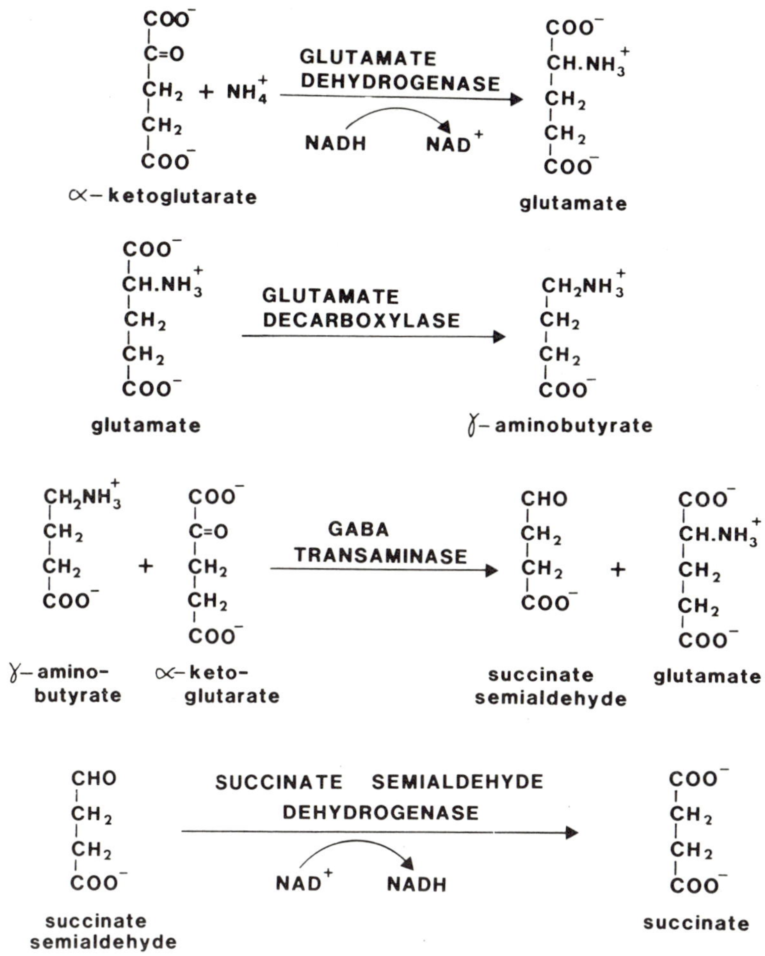

Figure 5.2 Reactions involved in the synthesis and degradation of GABA

5.1.2 γ-aminobutyrate changes in migraine

Welch *et al.*[2,3] reported that CSF levels of GABA were increased in all 28 of a series of cases of migraine examined during and shortly after attacks. They pointed out that CSF GABA levels were commonly raised soon after cerebral and brain stem infarction or ischaemia, and suggested that therefore the CSF GABA changes in migraine might be consequences of brain ischaemia. Dalessio[4] agreed with this suggestion.

We have not traced other observations on CSF GABA in migraine. Observations on blood GABA, part of which seems to originate from intestinal bacterial activity, would be difficult to assess in relation to migraine.

5.1.3 Interpretation of γ-aminobutyrate changes in migraine

It seems likely that the interpretation that Welch *et al.*[2,3] proferred is correct, in other words that raised CSF GABA levels in migraine are simply a consequence of cerebral ischaemia (or some other type of temporary cerebral injury). This interpretation at first sight would seem to carry the implication that cerebral ischaemia is invariably present in migraine since these investigators found CSF GABA changes in all the cases they studied. Such a conclusion would appear at variance with the cerebral blood flow studies of Olesen, Tfelt-Hansen *et al.*[5]. The reconciliation of this apparent conflict may lie in the comment of Welch *et al.*[3] that, because of their known interest in vascular disorder, they may have had referred to them a group of migraineurs who posed diagnostic problems. Thus the cases they studied may have been mainly, or entirely, of the classical type, and may have had more severe disturbances of neural function than do typical cases. If so, this could explain the apparent discrepancy between the frequency of ischaemic effects on brain metabolism found in Welch's population, and the evidences of ischaemia in the studies by the Danish cerebral blood flow workers.

The raised CSF GABA levels in migraine may simply be a consequence of cerebral ischaemia, which presumably interferes with GABA storage, re-uptake or metabolism. However it may not necessarily be the case that this escape of GABA into the CSF is itself without consequence. In view of the observations of Kelly *et al.*[1], the raised CSF GABA levels might have a local vasodilating effect which could conceivably reduce the postulated cerebral cortical ischaemia of migraine.

The question may be raised: could the increased CSF GABA levels simply reflect neurogenic inhibition in an area of cortex, much as in Leão's spreading depression, and not be a consequence of ischaemia? At present no validly based answer is available.

5.2 LACTATE

5.2.1 Biology

Lactate ($CH_3.CHOH.COO^-$) is a metabolic intermediate at the terminal stage of Embden-Meyerhof anaerobic glycolysis. It is formed by the reduction of pyruvate which, in the presence of sufficient available oxygen, is also converted to acetate which is then metabolised to CO_2 and water in the Krebs cycle. The formation of lactate in essence appears a blind-ended metabolic diversion to 'mop-up' pyruvate which cannot enter the Krebs cycle because sufficient O_2 is not available. Because the pyruvate – lactate reaction is reversible, should O_2 subsequently become available before irreparable consequences occur, the lactate can be reconverted to pyruvate for further metabolism. The formation of lactate from pyruvate also allows the oxidation of $NADH_2$ to NAD^+, which somewhat remotely facilitates continuing mitochondrial oxidation in the electron transport chain. It is generally accepted that increased lactate concentrations tend to correlate with effects of hypoxia or ischaemia. CSF and blood lactate concentrations behave as semi-independent variables[6].

5.2.2 Lactate changes in migraine

Skinhoj[7] examined the CSF lactate content in ten persons with common migraine. The level was raised in all (mean 2.14 ± 0.58 mmol/l, with normal values of 1.54 ± 0.16 mmol/l). The CSF HCO_3^- level was reduced (19.7 ± 2.3, as compared with a control value of 23.6 ± 0.09 mmol/l).

5.2.3 Interpretation of lactate changes in migraine

The raised CSF lactate levels may be due to cerebral hypoxia, or diminished Krebs cycle activity, during migraine. Possibly the changes are simply a consequence of ischaemia. It is possible that the CSF lactic acidosis of migraine may cause increased cerebral blood flow in subsequent stages of migraine attacks.

5.3 CYCLIC ADENOSINE MONOPHOSPHATE (cAMP)

5.3.1 Biology

Cyclic adenosine monophosphate is a so-called intracellular 'second messenger'. Its synthesis from adenosine triphosphate (ATP) is activated by the interaction of a number of different ligands with their respective cellular receptors, for example the binding of adrenaline or noradrenaline with the β-type of adrenoreceptor or of dopamine with its D_1 type receptors. The ligand – receptor interaction causes the enzyme adenylate cyclase to catalyse cAMP formation (Figure 5.3). In some instances the enzyme may be the actual receptor for the ligand. The cAMP so formed mediates a variety of intracellular metabolic activities in different types of cell.

Cyclic AMP is subsequently degraded to adenosine monophosphate (AMP) in a reaction catalysed by the enzyme phosphodiesterase. In many tissues cAMP seems to stimulate the activity of a protein kinase, thus leading to further molecular events.

Measurable concentrations of cAMP occur in plasma, and appear related to β-adrenoceptor stimulation, correlating better with plasma adrenaline than with plasma noradrenaline concentrations. The nucleotide also occurs in CSF.

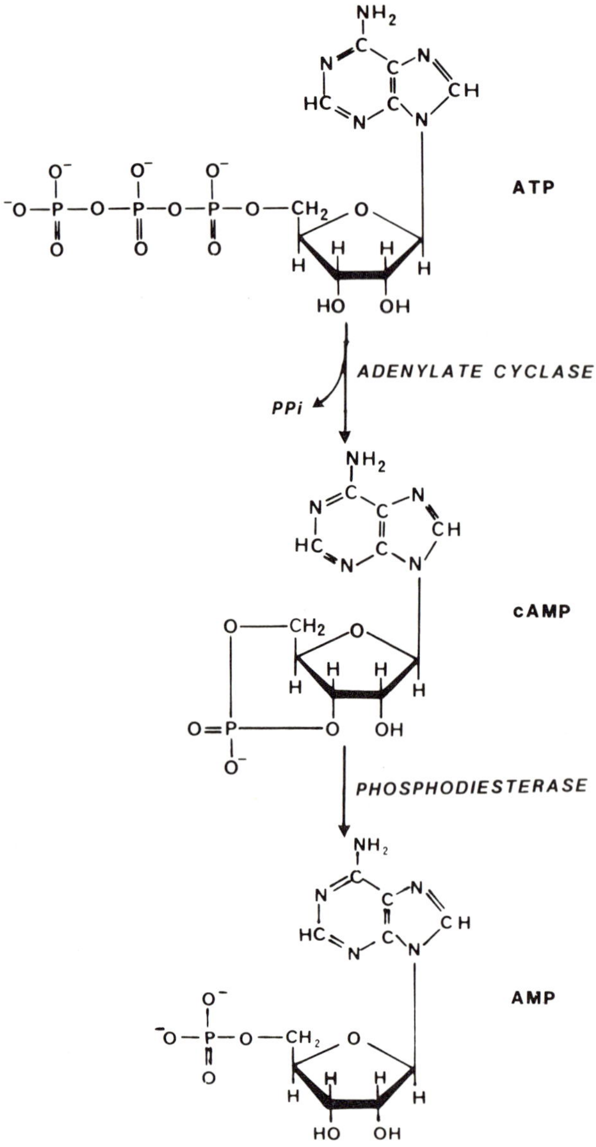

Figure 5.3 Cyclic AMP formation and degradation

5.3.2 Cyclic AMP changes in migraine

Welch *et al.*[2,3] reported raised cAMP levels in CSF during migraine attacks in the subjects whom they studied, probably a rather highly selected group (see

Section 5.2). Anthony[8,9] noted a mean increase of over 100% in plasma cAMP levels during migraine attacks in nine out of a series of ten subjects.

5.3.3 Interpretation of cAMP changes in migraine

Welch *et al.*[2,3] took the view that the raised cAMP levels they found during migraine attacks were simply a consequence of neural tissue ischaemia, like the simultaneous changes in CSF γ-aminobutyrate levels that they described. There seems no particular reason to disagree with this interpretation. Anthony[8,9] regarded the raised plasma cAMP levels he reported in migraine as a result of increased sympathetic nervous system activity, of which other evidences, for example raised plasma noradrenaline and dopamine-β-hydroxylase levels (see Sections 3.2 and 3.3), were also available. Again, the explanation appears reasonable in view of the knowledge that circulating catecholamines cause increased cAMP levels in plasma, at least in rats[10].

5.4 OTHER ADENINE NUCLEOTIDES

Rydzewski and Wachowicz[11] reported a comparison of platelet contents of adenosine triphosphate and adenosine diphosphate in 15 migraineurs and 12 control subjects. Nucleotide levels were measured both during and between migraine attacks. Migraineurs had been untreated for at least 1 week before the study. Levels of both nucleotides were increased in the migraineurs' platelets, both in and between headache attacks. The two adenosine nucleotides are intimately related metabolically, the diphosphate combining with inorganic phosphate to form the triphosphate in the process of oxidative phosphorylation which occurs at several stages along the ubquitous mitochondrial electron transport pathway. Adenosine triphosphate serves as a source of energy for many biochemical reactions. Rydzewski and Wachowicz[11] were uncertain as to the interpretation of the raised ADP and ATP levels in their migraineurs' platelets though the finding was consistent with these platelets being capable of greater metabolic activity than the platelets of control subjects. ADP in plasma, of course, is a potent platelet aggregating agent.

$$\text{ADP} + \text{Pi} \xrightleftharpoons{\substack{\text{ADENOSINE} \\ \text{TRIPHOSPHATASE}}} \text{ATP}$$

Burnstock[12] pointed out that ATP is a potent dilator of cerebral vessels, and also stimulates pain nerve endings. He proposed that it might have a role in the pathogenesis of migraine, perhaps being released from tissues as the result of ischaemia in earlier stages of the evolution of attacks.

5.5 ENKEPHALINS AND ENDORPHINS

The endorphins (endogenous morphine-like factors) and the enkephalins (biologically-active oligopeptide endorphin fractions) are newly recognised groups of substances whose role in migraine has begun to be explored. Nearly all knowledge in this area is comparatively recent and information has accumulated rapidly. Therefore the situation relating to these substances in migraine is a little difficult to assess.

5.5.1 Biology

Bloom[13] has provided a recent brief review of the topic.

5.5.1.1 Chemistry and formation

Various subfractions of β-lipotropin, a pituitary polypeptide, itself comprising a sequence of 90 aminoacids (Figure 5.4), possess biological activity. These peptide subfractions include three endorphins: α-endorphin (aminoacid sequence 61–76), γ-endorphin (aminoacids 61–77) and β-endorphin (aminoacids 61–91). A pentapeptide sequence common to all three endorphins (aminoacids 61–65) is also biologically active and is termed Met^5-enkephalin. It comprises the aminoacid sequence:

tyrosine-glycine-glycine-phenylalanine-methionine

A second enkephalin, Leu^5-enkephalin differs from Met^5-enkephalin only in replacement of methionine by leucine in the pentapeptide aminoacid sequence at its C-terminal. It is also biologically active.

tyr-	gly-	gly-	phe-	met-	thr-	ser-	glu-	lys-	ser-
61	62	63	64	65	66	67	68	69	70
gln-	thr-	pro-	leu-	val-	thr-	leu-	phe-	lys-	asn-
71	72	73	74	75	76	77	78	79	80
ala-	ile-	val-	lys-	asn-	ala-	his-	lys-	lys-	gly
81	82	83	84	85	86	87	88	89	90

Figure 5.4 The terminal 30 aminoacid sequence of β-lipotropin

Although the pentapeptide sequence of Met^5-enkephalin is contained within all three endorphins there are reasons for doubting that this enkephalin does arise in nature from the endorphins[14]. Its distribution and concentration in the brain does not parallel that of its postulated precursor, β-endorphin. Further, there are at least two known putative precursors for Leu^5-enkephalin that have been found in brain. These are the larger enkephalins α-neoendorphin and dynorphin (Figure 5.5) which are as potent as Leu^5-enkephalin, which is suspected of being an (?artefactual) cleavage product of the larger oligopeptides. Additionally, potential precursor polypeptides for Met^5-enkephalin, apart from the endorphins, have been located in adrenal chromaffin cells and in the striatum.

α-neoendorphin : tyr-gly-gly-phe-leu-arg-lys--

dynorphin : tyr-gly-gly-phe-leu-arg-arg--

Figure 5.5 Aminoacid sequences in α-neoendorphin and dynorphin

Recent studies indicate that β-endorphin is itself part of the aminoacid sequence of a giant polypeptide (molecular weight 31 000 daltons), termed 'pro-opio-melanocortin'. This macromolecule contains the peptide sequences of β-lipotropin (of which β-endorphin is a part), corticotrophin and α-, β-, and γ-melanocyte stimulating hormones.

5.5.1.2 Occurrence

Enkephalin activity (exactly which enkephalin is often not certain because of lack of specificity of current cytochemical assays) occurs in many parts of the nervous system, with highest levels in the striatum, pallidum, hippocampus, thalamus, periaqueductal grey matter and substantia gelatinosa of the spinal cord. The enkephalins occur within short axon interneurons which may form presynaptic axo-axonic synapses on neurons of other functional systems.

The major endorphin in the nervous system is the β-type. This is present at high concentration in the pituitary (in the intermediate lobe and corticotrophs of the anterior lobe). It also occurs in neurons of the basomedial and basolateral hypothalamus which project to the anterior hypothalamus, septum, periaqueductal grey matter and pons (including the locus coeruleus [15]). The distribution of pro-opio-melanocortin is similar to that of β-endorphin.

Enkephalin and endorphin-like activity in CSF and blood can be measured with radioimmunoassay techniques though, as indicated above, individual enkephalins may not be recognised specifically. The β-endorphin in plasma probably originates in the pituitary[16]. CSF endogenous opioid levels are increased in the presence of pain and of emotion, during acupuncture and in schizophrenia: stress can cause the pituitary to release β-endorphin[17]. Serum β-endorphin levels increase in pregnancy.

5.5.1.3 Effects

There appear to be several types of endorphin receptors (e.g.μ, κ, s types) but, at the time of writing, their classification does not appear settled.

Enkephalins and β-endorphin depress naloxone-sensitive neurons in most regions (naloxone is a specific opiate antagonist). However in the hippocampus this effect so disinhibits neurons with a normal inhibitory function that the overall regional consequence is hyperexcitability. The effect of β-endorphin is more prolonged than that of the enkephalins. Enkephalins and β-endorphins all produce analgesia when introduced into the nervous system. Their other effects are still being explored.

5.5.2 Endorphin and enkephalin changes in migraine

There are both experimental data and a number of lines of speculation regarding endorphins and enkephalins in migraine.

5.5.2.1 *Observations*

Anselmi *et al.*[17] reported decreased levels of enkephalins in CSF during attacks of migraine (ten subjects), as compared with the headache-free periods (eight subjects) in which values resembled those for control subjects. Cerebrospinal fluid enkephalin levels were found to be unmeasurably low in five cluster headache sufferers, when headache free. At the end of migraine attacks there was a rise in mean serum β-endorphin-like immunoreactivity, though in the headache-free period activity was similar to that in control subjects. Appenzeller *et al.*[18] found no alteration in serum β-endorphin activity in attacks of common migraine in four cases. Facchinetti *et al.*[19] reported serum lipotropin and β-endorphin levels in eight control subjects, 11 'daily headache' and 11 common migraine sufferers. In the three groups mean β-lipotropin levels were, respectively 83.6 ± 13.1, 57.6 ± 9.5 and 75.3 ± 12.0 pmol/l, and β-endorphin levels 26.0 ± 6.1, 16.8 ± 2.5 and 24.4 ± 5.8 pmol/l under basal conditions. Traditional Chinese acupuncture raised the β-lipotropin and β-endorphin levels in the control subjects only. Baldi *et al.*[16] found that in 26 migraineurs' plasma β-endorphin levels fell from a mean of 11.2 ± 1.4 pmol/l (controls 12.6 ± 1.3) to a mean of 5.3 ± 0.5 pmol/l during migraine attacks.

Thus plasma (or serum) β-endorphin levels in migraineurs appeared normal between headaches in all three reported studies, but fell during migraine attacks in the study of Baldi *et al.*[16], and appeared to rise towards the end of attacks in the investigation of Anselmi *et al.*[17] and as reported by Della Bella *et al.*[20] (in what may be the same study). It is difficult to be sure whether these apparently conflicting results represent a genuine difference (which must be recociled in the future) or are a consequence of measurements at different stages in the evolution of migraine attacks.

Centonze *et al.*[21] reported two patients in whom intravenous administration of the opiate antagonist naloxone relieved the neurological deficits of migraine, but not the headache. It is known that naloxone can temporarily reverse ischaemic neurological defects, and morphine can exaggerate them[22].

5.5.2.2 *Hypotheses*

Sicuteri[23] drew attention to the progressive rise in plasma β-endorphin levels that occurs during pregnancy. He suggested that, because of the analgesic effect of this peptide, this rise might explain why migraine tended to lessen in pregnancy. He considered the plasma β-endorphin originated in the pituitary, but wondered if it might also be produced by the placenta. Anselmi *et al.*[17] raised the possibility that circulating β-endorphin might affect the central nervous system by back diffusion, presumably into the hypothalamus. Later Sicuteri[24] stated that the drug captopril was an effective migraine prophylactic. as captopril inhibits various peptidases which catalyse the breakdown of enkephalins and endorphin. Sicuteri proposed that the drug might benefit migraine by increasing endogenous opioid concentrations. He also proceeded[25] to point out that morphine was not as effective in migraine as would be expected, and on this basis suggested that migraine might represent the consequence of a genetic or spontaneous impairment of the neural endorphin system. He further developed this idea[26], and stated that CSF met[5]-enkephalin levels were reduced in migraine attacks. He related migraine to a 'quasimorphine abstinence syndrome'. In migraine he proposed that there was a deficiency of the endogenous opioid system with neurotransmitter storage 'incontinence' in opioid-dependent neurons. Agnoli *et al.*[15] devised a rather detailed hypothetical scheme to explain migraine in terms of altered endogenous opioid function. They suggested that endogenous opioid activity, which modulates function of the locus coeruleus, becomes reduced in migraine. This allows the locus coeruleus to initiate release of amines. The amine release causes vasoconstriction (presumably by acting via the pathways already discussed – Section 2.3) and thus initiates the clinical migraine mechanism.

5.5.3 Interpretation of endorphin and enkephalin changes in migraine

The decreased CSF enkephalin levels reported during migraine could reflect failure of a pain dampening element in central neurotransmission, and thus represent a significant component of the migraine mechanism. However, the changes might also simply represent a consequence of the cerebral circulatory alterations of migraine, and perhaps of brain ischaemia. If the time course of the CSF enkephalin changes were known the situation might be easier to interpret, but at this stage there is not sufficient information to permit soundly based deductions.

In the present state of knowledge the changes in circulating β-endorphin during migraine are probably best interpreted as reflecting altered pituitary function. Again, there are no clear data as to the time course of these changes relative to the time course of migraine attacks. Therefore it is difficult to know whether the changes correlate with some primary, perhaps causative molecular mechanism, whether they represent consequences of cerebral circulatory alterations in migraine, or whether they are simply a response to the 'stress' of migraine. Stress does raise plasma β-endorphin levels[17]. To argue that a fall in circulating β-endorphin would represent a fall in β-endorphin in the neural pathway mediating pain transmission appears of doubtful propriety, particularly when β-endorphin neurons are not known to be involved in the function of this pathway. To argue that decreased circulating β-endorphin would facilitate pain, or that an increase in the concentration of this oligopeptide in the circulation would help prevent migraine in pregnancy, ignores the question of how circulating β-endorphin would traverse the blood – brain barrier to reach synapses in the pain pathway. If we knew what happened to CSF β-endorphin during the various stages of migraine attacks, the latter line of argument might appear rather more tenable.

The findings of Centonze *et al.*[21] that the opiate antagonist naloxone may reverse the neurological deficits of migraine opens the possibility for a different role for opioids in the disorder. Perhaps opioids are concerned with the production of focal brain dysfunction, and relate to the aura mechanism.

The various hypotheses mentioned above (Section 5.5.2) concerning the role of the endogenous opioid system in migraine appear highly speculative reltive to the relatively insubstantial bulk of the available experimental data. The hypotheses, or parts of them, may be valid but proof is at present lacking.

5.6 TAURINE

Taurine is a sulphur-containing aminoacid which is a precursor for the bile acid taurocholic acid. In the body taurine appears to be derived from cysteine via cysteinesulphinic acid and hypotaurine (Figure 5.6)

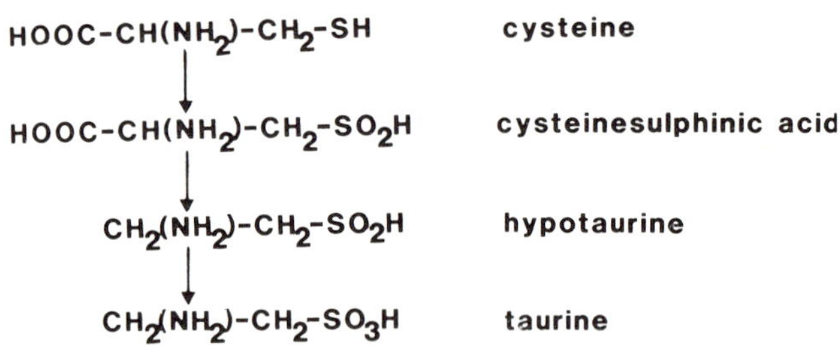

Figure 5.6 Derivation of taurine in the body

In the nervous system taurine exerts an inhibitory action, though whether it acts as an neurotransmitter or a neuromodulator remains uncertain. Cysteine is present in CSF and plasma (in the latter at a mean level of 60 μmol/l).

Dhopesh and Baskin[27] measured platelet taurine content in seven migraineurs during headaches and in the post-ictal phase. During attacks the mean taurine content was 0.172 ± 0.017 nmol/10^3 platelets/ml plasma, and this value fell to a mean of 0.129 ± 0.017 post-ictally. Using a one-tail *t*-test, the change was statistically significant ($p < 0.01$). Bearing in mind the well-documented fall in platelet serotonin content during migraine attacks, the authors speculated that during the attacks the taurine might have been taken up by platelets in place of serotonin. Platelets normally have a high content of taurine, most of which is probably acquired by uptake from plasma[28]. Whether the suggestion of Dhopesh and Baskin[27] is valid, and whether taurine could play any more active role in migraine, remain unknown.

5.7 CORTISOL

5.7.1 Biology

Cortisol (hydrocortisone) is the main hormone secreted by the adrenal cortex. Its secretion follows a diurnal rhythm with peak plasma concentrations occurring in the morning. Circulating levels increase in response to stress.

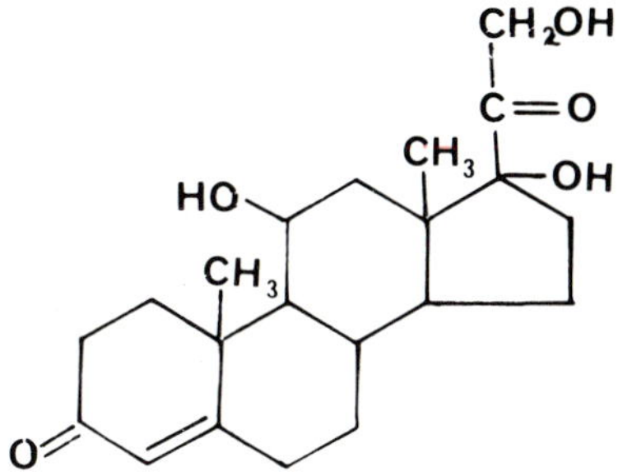

cortisol

Cortisol possesses both glucocorticoid and mineralocorticoid properties. It has anti-inflammatory effects, raises blood pressure and blood glucose levels and causes salt and water retention. Excess adrenal cortisol secretion produces the manifestations of Cushing's syndrome.

The clearance of cortisol is largely metabolic, the pathways of metabolism being as described by Cope[29]. Circulating plasma cortisol levels are usually in the range 10–25 μg/dl.

5.7.2 Cortisol changes in migraine

Ziegler *et al.*[30] stated that plasma cortisol levels were abnormally high, or showed aberrant peaks, in 64% of migraine attacks.

5.7.3 Interpretation of plasma cortisol changes in migraine

The plasma cortisol changes in migraine may be merely a consequence of stress. However, they could be related to the salt and water retention that occurs in some migraine attacks (see Section 6.1). Knowledge of the time course of plasma cortisol changes in attacks might clarify the role of the steroid in these circumstances.

References

1. Kelly, P.A.T., Grome, J.J. and McCulloch, J. (1981). Cerebrovascular and metabolic influences of GABA in relation to migraine. In Rose, F.C. and Zilkha, K.J. (eds.). *Progress in Migraine Research.* London: Pitman, 100–105
2. Welch, K.M.A., Chabi, E., Nell, J.H., Bartosh, K., Chee, A.N.C., Mathew, N.T. and Achar,

V.S. (1976). Biochemical comparison of migraine and stroke. *Headache,* **16,** 160–167

3. Welch, K.M.A., Chabi, E., Nell, J., Bartosh, K., Meyer, J.S. and Mathew, N.T. (1978). Similarities in biochemical effects of cerebral ischaemia in patients with cerebrovascular disease and migraine. In Greene, R. (ed.). *Current Concepts in Migraine Research.* New York: Raven Press, 1–9
4. Dalessio, D.J. (1979). Classification and mechanism of migraine. *Headache,* **19,** 114–120
5. Olesen, J., Tfelt-Hansen, P., Henricksen, L. and Larsen, B. (1981). The common migraine attack may not be initiated by cerebral ischaemia. *Lancet,* **2,** 438–440
6. Posner, J.B. and Plum, F. (1967). Independence of blood and cerebrospinal fluid lactate. *Archives of Neurology,* **16,** 492–496
7. Skinhoj, E. (1973). Hemodynamic studies within the brain during migraine. *Archives of Neurology,* **29,** 95–98
8. Anthony, M. (1981). Biochemical indices of sympathetic activity in migraine. *Cephalalgia,* **1,** 83–89
9. Anthony, M. (1982). Serotonin and cyclic nucleotides in migraine. *Advances in Neurology,* **33,** 45–49
10. Kunitada, S. Honna, M. and Ui, M. (1978). Increase in plasma cyclic AMP dependent on endogenous catecholamines. *European Journal of Pharmacology,* **48,** 159–169
11. Rydzewski, W. and Washowicz, B. (1978). Adenine nucleotides in platelets in and between migraine attacks. In Green, R. (ed.). *Current Concepts in Migraine Research.* New York: Raven Press, 153–158
12. Burnstock, G. (1981). Pathophysiology of migraine: a new hypothesis. *Lancet,* **1,** 1397–1398
13. Bloom, F.E. (1983). The endorphins: a growing family of pharmacologically pertinent peptides. *Annual Review of Pharmacology and Toxicology,* **23,** 151–170
14. Cooper, J.R., Bloom, F.E. and Roth, R.H. (1982). *The Biochemical Basis of Neuropharmacology.* New York: Oxford University Press, 4th Edition
15. Agnoli, A., Denaro, A., Ceci, E. and Falaschi, P. (1982). On the etiopathogenesis of migraine: a possible link between the amines and endorphin hypothesis. *Advances in Neurology,* **33,** 99–106
16. Baldi, E., Salmon, S., Anselmi, B., Spillantini, M.G., Cappelli, G., Brocchi, A. and Sicuteri, F. (1982). Intermittent hypoendorphinaemia in migraine attack. *Cephalalgia,* **2,** 77–81
17. Anselini, B., Baldi, E., Casacci, F. and Salmon, S. (1980). Endogenous opioids in cerebrospinal fluid and blood in idiopathic headache sufferers. *Headache,* **20,** 294–299
18. Appenzeller, O., Atkinson, R.A. and Standefer, J.C. (1981). Serum-β-endorphin in cluster headache and common migraine. In Rose, F.C. and Zilkha, K.J. (eds.). *Progress in Migraine Research. 1.* London: Pitman, 106–109
19. Facchinetti, F., Nappi, G., Savoldi, F. and Genazzani, A.R. (1981). Primary headaches: reduced circulating β-lipotropin and β-endorphin levels with impaired reactivity of acupuncture. *Cephalalgia,* **1,** 195–201
20. Della Bella, D., Carenzi, A., Casacci, F., Anselmi, B., Baldi, E. and Salmon, S. (1982). Enorphins in the pathogenesis of headache. In Critchley, M., Friedman, A.P., Gorini, S. and Sicuteri, F. (eds.). Headache: Physiopathological and Clinical Concepts. *Advances in Neurology,* **33,** 75–79
21. Centonze, V., Brucoli, C., Macinagrossa, G., Attolini, E., Campanozzi, F. and Albano, O. (1983). Non-familial hemiplegic migraine responsive to naloxone. *Cephalalgia,* **3,** 125–127
22. Baskin, D.S. and Hosobuchi, Y. (1981). Naloxone reversal of ischaemic neurological deficits in man. *Lancet,* **2,** 272– 275
23. Sicuteri, F. (1980). Opioids, pregnancy and the disappearance of headache. *Headache,* **20,** 220–221
24. Sicuteri, F. (1981). Enkephalinase inhibition relieves pain syndromes of central dysnociocep-tion (migraine and related headache). *Cephalalgia,* **1,** 229–232
25. Sicuteri, F. (1981). Opioid receptor impairment – underlying mechanism in 'pain disease'? *Cephalalgia,* **1,** 77–82
26. Sicuteri, F. (1982). Natural opioids in migraine. In Critchley, M., Friedman, A.P., Gorini, S. and Sicuteri, F. (eds.) Headache: Physiopathological and Clinical Concepts. *Advances in Neurology,* **33,** 65–74
27. Dhopesh, V.P. and Baskin, S.I. (1982). Change in platelet taurine and migraine. *Headache,* **22,** 165–166

28. Da Prada, M., Richards, J.G. and Ketti, R. (1981). Amine storage organelles in platelets. In Gordon, J.L. (ed.). *Platelets in Biology and Pathology-2.* Amsterdam: Elsevier, 107–145
29. Cope, C.L. (1972). *Adrenal Steroids and Disease.* London: Pitman. 2nd edition
30. Ziegler, D.K., Hassanein, R.S., Kodanaz, A. and Meek. J.C. (1979). Circadian rhythms of plasma cortisol in migraine. *Journal of Neurology, Neurosurgery and Psychiatry,* **42,** 741–748

6

Biochemical changes that are difficult to classify, or speculative

For a variety of reasons, certain biochemical changes reported in migraine do not fit easily into the foregoing categories of changes which appear part of the migraine mechanism or consequences of the mechanism. These biochemical alterations, whose relationship to the migraine mechanism is difficult to categorise in that some appear consequences of what could be seen as a migraine precursor disturbance, while some are unsupported by studies in migraine, are dealt with below.

6.1 WATER, ELECTROLYTES AND RELATED HORMONES

6.1.1 Changes reported

Alterations in fluid balance are known to occur in relation to some migraine attacks. Pfeiffer *et al.*[1] measured plasma protein levels and the haematocrit during migraine attacks, and after treatment of attacks. Protein concentrations and the haematocrit both decreased after treatment, suggesting that the blood volume was decreased during the headache.

Campbell *et al.*[2] studied fluid balance in 26 migraine sufferers and eight control subjects. They noted that some persons with migraine developed oedema before their headaches. There was a 5–6% decrease in plasma protein content before, during and after the attacks. Mean plasma sodium content was 349 mg% in the prodromal phase, 359 mg% during the attacks and 333 mg% after the attack, with the mean sodium content subsequently rising to its basal value of 339 mg%. These workers also studied the effects of a water load in migraine sufferers. The volume of the induced diuresis did not differ between migraine sufferers and controls, but there was a greater urinary excretion of Cl^- in the migraine sufferers. Na^+ excretion at rest did not differ between the migraineurs and the controls, but increased considerably in migraineurs, but not in the controls, during the diuresis. On this basis Campbell *et al.*[2] concluded that there was fluid retention before and during migraine in the average patient. There was also an altered urinary electrolyte response to induced diuresis, as compared with controls. Thus Campbell *et al.*[2] came to a contrary conclusion to Pfeiffer *et al.*[1] about body fluid volume during migraine. Ostfeld *et al.*[3] noted a gain in weight commencing 4 hours to 6 days before the onset of headache in 48 of 51 migraineurs. Diuresis developed as the headache eased. In these subjects use of a diuretic failed to prevent the migraine attacks. The findings were generally in keeping with those of Campbell *et al.*[2]. Schottstaedt and Wolff[4] followed daily urine volume and urinary Na^+, K^+ and creatinine excretions in a group of ten migraineurs who experienced 28 attacks during the study period. Mean urine volumes, Na^+, K^+ and creatinine excretions were all decreased before or in the early stages of migraine, as compared with these parameters in the phase of subsiding headaches. In 63 out of 134 patients weight gain and fluid retention occurred before attacks, sometimes beginning up to a few days prior to the headache. Pre-headache weight gain was not uniformly present, nor was post-headache weight loss and diuresis. In subjects who had pre-migraine weight gain, giving a diuretic did not prevent headache, despite the production of a diuresis. Inducing water retention by administering pitressin or desoxycortisterone did not induce migraine.

After these studies some three decades ago the question of water retention in migraine appears to have been little investigated. This apparent neglect may have occurred because the failure of induced diuresis to prevent expected migraine attacks suggested that the fluid changes were not part of the causative mechanism of the disorder, and therefore not a rewarding subject for study. However Brainard[5] found that 1 gram of NaCl induced attacks in 14 out of 15 migraineurs, while intake of placebo was followed by an attack in only 1 out of 10 subjects. The NaCl load caused raised plasma angiotensin levels. Horthe *et al.*[6] stated that plasma aldosterone levels were abnormal in two migrainous subjects whom they studied, though levels of the steroid were not greatly increased at the time of migraine attacks.

6.1.2 Interpretation of water and electrolyte changes in migraine

The frequency with which fluid and electrolyte changes occur before and during migraine attacks suggests that these changes reflect some basic migraine mechanism. Induced diuresis consistently fails to prevent expected migraine attacks (and this must be a matter confirmed by the personal experiences of many neurologists). Therefore the fluid and electrolyte changes in migraine seem to be a by-product of the causative biochemical changes of the disorder, and not directly related causally to the production of the headaches. It would seem likely that the fluid retention is due to hormonal changes, which may conceivably be secondary to altered hypothalamic activity. Adequate data do not appear to exist which would allow this possibility to be evaluated – for example measurements of simultaneous plasma concentrations of antidiuretic hormone, aldosterone, Na^+, K^+, Cl^-, and urinary excretions of H_2O, Na^+, K^+ and Cl^-. Investigation of these matters, using contemporary analytical methods, should be capable of determining why water retention may begin several days prior to migraine attacks. This information, in turn, should illuminate one of the earliest, or even the earliest, disturbance that may be part of migraine. This knowledge might lead the way to exploring the true initiating biochemical events of migraine.

6.2 AMMONIUM

In a pilot study of 22 adults with migraine Bruyn *et al.*[7] reported raised blood ammonium concentrations (mean 103 μg%, compared with a mean value of 40 μg% for normal subjects). It was not completely clear whether the measurements were taken during or between attacks. It is very difficult to interpret this finding, and there do not appear to have been subsequent reports on the matter.

6.3 SUBSTANCE P

There have been suggestions from time to time that this peptide neurotransmitter may be involved in the pathogenesis of migraine. However, so far as we are aware, there is no evidence of altered substance P function in migraine attacks.

6.3.1 Biology

Substance P is an oligopeptide containing the following sequence of 11 aminoacids (Figure 6.1)

arginine
|
proline
|
lysine
|
proline
|
glutamine
|
glutamine
|
phenylalanine
|
phenylalanine
|
glycine
|
leucine
|
methionine-NH_2

Figure 6.1 Sequence of aminoacids in substance P

A recent account of its biology is available[8]. Substance P is found in small neurons in many parts of the nervous system, but particularly in the substantia gelatinosa of the spinal cord where it is a possible excitatory neurotransmitter or, more probably, a neuromodulator[9] for incoming sensory impulses conveying pain information. The oligopeptide also occurs at higher concentrations in the striatum and substantia nigra, the amygdaloid, hypothalamus and cerebral cortex. Together with serotonin, it is present in neurons that project from the mid-brain raphe to the spinal cord. Its more detailed role in neural events is still to be clarified.

6.3.2 Possible role in migraine

There have been suggestions that an excessive localised release of substance P may facilitate pain impulse transmission from one side of the head during migraine attacks and also that substance P and other neurotransmitter oligopeptides present in facial nerve fibres may, after release at nerve terminals, contribute to the extracranial vascular events of migraine[10]. In the present state of knowledge, these suggestions appear purely attempts to incriminate substance P in migraine by virtue of its having a distribution in the body which could allow it to play a role in the disorder. Unfortunately there is no evidence beyond this.

References

1. Pfeiffer, C., Dreisbach, R.H., Roby, C.C. and Glass, H.G. (1943). Etiology of the migraine syndrome: a physiological approach. *Journal of Laboratory and Clinical Medicine,* **28,** 1219–1225
2. Campbell, D.A., Hay, K.M. and Tonks, E.M. (1951). An investigation of the salt and water balance in migraine. *British Medical Journal,* **2,** 1424–1429
3. Ostfeld, A.M., Reis, D.J., Goodell, H. and Wolff, H.G. (1955). Headache and hydration. The significance of two varieties of fluid accumulation in patients with vascular headache of the migraine type. *Archives of Internal Medicine,* **96,** 142–152
4. Schottstaedt, W.W. and Wolff, H.G. (1955). Variations in fluid and electrolyte excretion in association with vascular headache of the migraine type. *Archives of Neurology and Psychiatry,* **73,** 158–164
5. Brainard, J.B. (1981). Angiotensin and aldosterone elevation in salt-induced migraine. *Headache,* **21,** 222– 226
6. Horthe, C.E., Wainscott, G., Neylan, C. and Wilkinson, M.I.P. (1975). Progesterone, oestradiol and aldosterone levels in plasma during the menstrual cycle of women suffering from migraine. *Journal of Endocrinology,* **65,** 24 P
7. Bruyn, G.W., Douma, G.J. and Gathier, J.C. (1971). Migraine and hyperammonaemia. In *Proceedings of the International Headache Symposium, Elsinore, Denmark.* Basel: Sandoz, 41–43
8. Iversen, L.L. (1983). Non opioid neuropeptides in mammalian CNS. *Annual Review of Pharmacology and Toxicology,* **23,** 1–27
9. Jessell, T.M. (1982). Neurotransmitters and CNS disease. Pain. *Lancet,* **2,** 1084–1088
10. Moskowitz, M.A., Reinhardt, J.F. Jr, Romero, J., Melamed, E. and Pettibone, D.J. (1979). Neurotransmitters and the fifth cranial nerve: is there a relation to the headache phase of migraine? *Lancet,* **2,** 883–885

7

Exogenous chemical substances that influence migraine

Various exogenous chemicals are known to influence migraine, either in a beneficial or a detrimental way. Thus certain drugs may relieve attacks of migraine that are already present, or prevent attacks developing, whilst other drugs and chemical agents appear to provoke attacks. By studying what is known of the mode of action of these substances it may be possible to gain further insights into the mechanisms of migraine pathogenesis.

For each substance to be considered, evidence will be considered as to (a) its effectiveness in relation to migraine; (b) its known mode or modes of action at the physiolological (tissue and organ) level; and (c) its known actions at the biochemical (molecular) level. These actions will then be interpreted in relation to possible mechanisms of migraine production.

Certain drugs useful in cluster headache rather than in migraine are also considered, in the hope that their mechanism of action in cluster headache may throw light on the molecular events of migraine as well as on the disorder for which they are used.

7.1 SUBSTANCES USED TO TREAT MIGRAINE ATTACKS

Current neurological practice employs a number of substances to treat migraine attacks. These substances include: (i) ergotamine and aspirin, both of which appear to have an effect of interrupting some fundamental component of the migraine mechanism; (ii) various non-steroidal anti- inflammatory agents which may have a specific antimigraine action, but whose efficacy in the disorder is not yet well established; (iii) certain weak and strong analgesics whose role appears to be pain suppression rather than interference with the more primary causative mechanisms of the disorder; (iv) antiemetics, which attempt to relieve only the symptoms of nausea and vomiting; and (v) sedatives, which seem to help the migraine sufferer largely by blunting his awareness or by affording him sleep during his time of suffering.

Of these substances, only ergotamine and aspirin appear likely to have a specific antimigraine role, and they will be the main ones considered here.

7.1.1 Ergotamine

The whole group of ergot alkaloids is the subject of a detailed monograph[1].

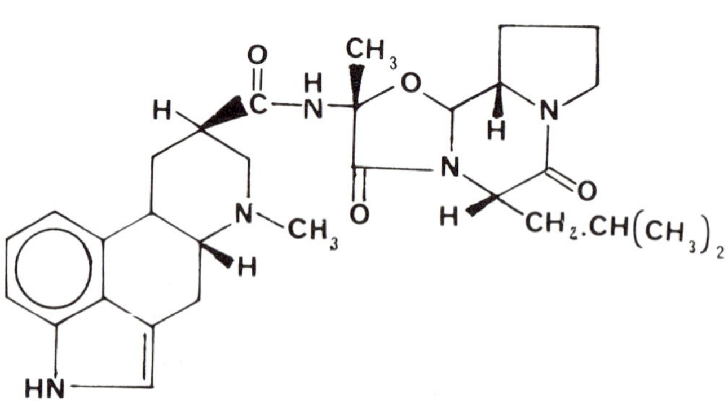

ergotamine

7.1.1.1 Clinical efficacy

Ergotamine has been used in treating migraine for a century. Initially it was given as a component of an alcoholic extract of ergot but, since its chemical isolation by Stoll in 1920, the pure substance has been available. The established clinical use of ergotamine thus antedates the contemporary technique of placebo-controlled double-blind clinical trial. The evidence of its efficacy in migraine is largely anecdotal, though based on the accumulated testimony of time.

Clinical experience makes it abundantly clear that ergotamine is far from efficacious in migraine, though it appears to be most effective when given parenterally. It is now realised that, in aqueous solution, ergotamine isomerises to a considerable extent to form a pharmacologically inactive epimer (ergotaminine). Therefore injections of the drug, unless freshly made up from pure ergotamine powder, usually deliver only about 50% of the nominal dose of the active substance. Further, if given by mouth, the drug is less than 2% bioavailable because of its extensive presystemic metabolism in the gut wall or liver or both. Thus there now appears to be adequate pharmacokinetic reason for the inconsistent effectiveness of orally-administered ergotamine[2]. Bearing this in mind, it is probably only the data from parenterally-administered ergotamine that should be taken as evidence of the efficacy of the drug in migraine. While this evidence is merely testimonial, it certainly suggests that ergotamine can relieve migraine headache. Clinical experience indicates that, the earlier ergotamine is taken during an attack of migraine, the greater the chance that it will provide pain relief.

Ergotamine has sometimes been used, with a measure of success, as a migraine prophylactic taken on a regular daily basis: it is certainly effective when used in this way in cluster headache prophylaxis. In general the regular use of ergotamine as a prophylactic in migraine is regarded as undesirable, for fear that it may cause rebound headache (Section 7.3.4). However, it should be noted that this problem does not appear to arise when the drug is taken two or three times a day in cluster headache attack prevention, though the period of administration in this circumstance may be shorter than that employed in migraine prophylaxis.

7.1.1.2 Actions at a physiological level

Ergotamine is a potent vasoconstrictor, at least on extracranial vessels[3], including veins[4]. It constricts scalp arterio-venous shunts[5-8], thus diverting extracranial blood flow into the scalp capillaries. In over-dosage it may produce profound peripheral vasoconstriction, endothelial damage and even gangrene. There is some evidence that it is not a constrictor of intracranial vessels[8] and at therapeutically effective doses, even in migraine attacks, it appears not to reduce cerebral blood flow[9-11].

Ergotamine can cause nausea (probably by an effect on the chemoreceptor trigger zone of the medulla) and cramping pain in skeletal muscles. It produces a degree of uterine contraction.

7.1.1.3 Actions at a molecular level

Blood vessels The classical interpretation of the mode of action of ergotamine is that the drug is an α-adrenoceptor agonist, and that this effect causes vasoconstriction. At supratherapeutic dosage it has a degree of competitive antagonist effect at α-receptors. Portions of the ergotamine molecule bears a steric resemblance to the molecule of serotonin. It is likely that an agonist type effect on vascular serotonin receptors causes, or at least contributes to, the vasoconstrictor effect of ergotamine[12-15]. However, ergotamine blocks the vasoconstrictor effect of administered serotonin[16]. Horowski[17] stated that ergotamine was also a central dopamine agonist.

Ergotamine does not seem to interfere with cerebral vascular prostaglandin synthesis, according to Gaudet *et al.*[18]. However, Spierings *et al.*[19] found that the drug (10^{-5} mol/l) did inhibit prostaglandin formation in rabbit ear vessels. This effect was thought to be due to inhibition of either of the enzymes phospholipase A_2 or cyclo-oxygenase[20].

Platelets Ergotamine also appears to act on platelet serotonin receptors. It inhibits thromboxane formation by human platelets[19], though possibly only at doses which would be toxic in humans[21].

7.1.1.4 Relation of drug action to the mechanism of migraine

The extracranial vasoconstrictor action of ergotamine, and the fact that it is more effective if taken early in the course of migraine attacks, fit with the type of hypothesis of migraine pathogenesis that sees the pain of the disorder as arising from distension of extracranial vessels. The effect of the drug on platelet serotonin receptors, and hence on platelet function, may explain how ergotamine could provide prophylaxis against migraine, and also interfere with the earliest stages of the mechanism of migraine attacks, if this mechanism involves platelet activation.

As yet, non-toxic doses of ergotamine appear to have no known clinical effect on human central nervous system function, except perhaps for causing vomiting. Therefore the known effectiveness of ergotamine in treating migraine attacks cannot readily be explained in terms of neural hypotheses of migraine production. Admittedly, ergotamine may act as a serotonin agonist at central serotoninergic synapses, though so far there appears to be no proof of this action at therapeutic drug concentrations in man. If this effect did apply, it could explain how ergotamine relieved migraine in terms of the hypothesis that the pain of the disorder arises from central nervous system serotonin depletion. However, if this mode of action did apply, ergotamine should relieve all types of pain, and not merely the pain of migraine, since it would be expected to influence all pain impulse transmission at synapses in the substantia gelatinosa. As far as we are aware, there is no evidence that ergotamine is a generally acting analgesic. Certainly it has not come into use for that purpose in clinical medicine.

Thus, in terms of contemporary knowledge, the effect of ergotamine in migraine fits much better with the vascular than the neural hypotheses of migraine pathogenesis.

7.1.2 Aspirin

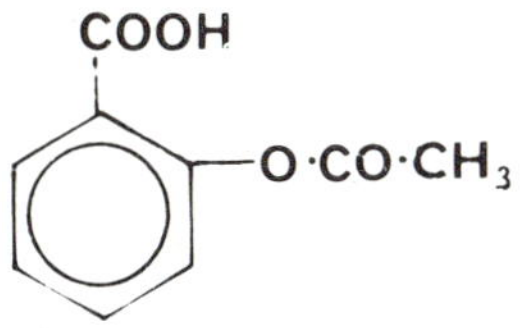

aspirin

7.1.2.1 Clinical efficacy

Aspirin has long been regarded as a household remedy for milder migraine. Until recently it had received little formal medical recognition as an effective therapy for the attacks, though there were certain exceptions (see,for example references[22,23]). However, a series of relatively recent studies from the Princess Margaret Migraine Clinic in London[24] has popularised the use of aspirin in treating attacks of the disorder. Many contemporary clinicians have come to regard the drug as almost equipotent to oral ergotamine in managing migraine attacks. We know of no placebo-controlled studies demonstrating the efficacy of aspirin in migraine. The basis for its use rests on the strength of clinical opinion rather than on the outcome of impeccably designed experimental studies. Ross Lee *et al.*[25], in analysing aspects of migraine which correlated with the ability of aspirin to relieve the headache, found that the presence of an aura during attacks was the only factor that seemed related to the benefit. Possibly the presence of an aura permitted patients to take aspirin earlier in the evolution of attacks than they would have if they had no warning of impending headache. In this same study it was also noted that, if aspirin did relieve migraine, only a comparatively low dose (600 mg orally in adults) was often required. These various observations indicated that a relatively small amount of aspirin, taken early in the evolution of migraine, had some chance of providing useful relief. Larger aspirin doses taken when headache was established appear to provide only limited relief. These findings suggest that aspirin may have a specific effect on the early stages of the migraine mechanism.

If this were so, one might predict that aspirin, taken on a regular basis, should prevent migraine. In a small but well-designed double-blind controlled trial, O'Neill and Mann[26] did demonstrate that aspirin (650 mg b.d.) had a migraine prophylactic effect. Masel *et al.*[27] noted similar benefit in their studies of migraine prophylaxis, but had used aspirin in conjunction with dipyridamole, so that the individual role of aspirin is impossible to assess. Ryan and Ryan[28] also found that regular aspirin prophylaxis decreased mean migraine frequency in patients. Other non-steroidal anti-inflammatory agents such as tolfenamic acid, have migraine-preventative effects[29].

7.1.2.2 Action at a physiological level

Aspirin is traditionally recognised as a mild analgesic which has antipyretic, anti-inflammatory and uricosuric actions. It has an antiplatelet action, inhibiting platelet aggregation, and this action may cause a degree of bleeding tendency.

In overdosage aspirin causes tinnitus and gastric irritation.

Amano and Meyer[30] showed that aspirin, in a single dose of 972 mg, caused slightly decreased cerebral blood flow in humans with vascular or non-vascular headaches. This action presumably occurs via inhibition of eicosanoid formation. Pickard *et al.*[31] showed that salicylate (not aspirin), at higher concentrations, lessened the cerebral blood flow increase which can be provoked by carbon dioxide inhalation.

7.1.2.3 Action at a biochemical level

It is necessary to draw a distinction between aspirin (acetylsalicylic acid) and its hydrolysis product salicylate. The latter is formed rapidly in the body after aspirin is absorbed, due to the catalytic activity of esterases in the gut wall, plasma and liver. Both aspirin and salicylate at therapeutic concentrations have one known mechanism of action which has been studied most extensively in platelets. In platelets aspirin inhibits aggregability and serotonin release[32]. Both aspirin and salicylate are thought to act on the enzyme cyclo-oxygenase[33], which catalyses the conversion of arachidonic acid to prostaglandin endoperoxides, though aspirin is very much the more efficient inhibitor of the enzyme. Aspirin and salicylate appear to have different modes of action on the platelet enzyme, and to act on it at slightly different intramolecular sites[34]. Aspirin appears to inhibit the cyclo-oxygenase of platelets irreversibly by acetylating serine residues on the active site of the enzyme. Since platelets cannot synthesise new cyclo-oxygenase, this inhibitory effect continues for the remainder of the life of the platelet. Salicylate appears to bind reversibly to the platelet enzyme, but not to inactivate it. However it may then impede to some extent the inhibitory action of aspirin on the enzyme. Aspirin is also said to inhibit irreversibly the endothelial cell cyclo-oxygenase whose activity results in prostacyclin formation. The duration of this effect is time- and aspirin-concentration dependent, since, unlike platelets, endothelial cells can synthesise new cyclo-oxygenase. Higher aspirin doses are reported as necessary to inhibit vessel wall as compared with platelet eicosanoid formation. Salicylate, even in high doses, has no direct inhibitory effect on endothelial cyclo-oxygenase but can diminish the effect of aspirin on vessel wall prostacyclin formation[35]. However, salicylate appears to have an effect in inhibiting cyclo-oxygenase somewhere in the body, since salicylate intake decreases urinary prostaglandin E_1 and E_2 metabolite excretion[36] and salicylate, administered as its sodium salt, affords relief in rheumatic disease.

The other therapeutic effects of aspirin (or of salicylate derived from it *in vivo*) may be related to cyclo-oxygenase inhibition, but the biochemical mechanisms of these effects do not appear to have been investigated in great detail.

Nor have the respective roles of unhydrolysed aspirin and salicylate been clarified in all circumstances.

In overdosage, salicylate uncouples oxidative phosphorylation, and impairs prothrombin formation.

7.1.2.4 Relation of drug action to the mechanisms of migraine

The circumstances in which aspirin appears most effective in migraine, in other words, when given early in the evolution of attacks – taken in conjunction with its only known biochemical mode of action, cyclo-oxygenase inhibition, suggest that the drug has its specific effect in migraine by interfering with eicosanoid formation early in the course of the disorder. Platelet aggregation, which involves thromboxane formation and release, occurs in migraine, and seems a likely point at which aspirin might interfere. Inhibition of platelet cyclo-oxygenase would also prevent the release of thromboxane A_2 and serotonin, substances which might contribute to the vascular spasm of migraine. Minimising this spasm might reduce endothelial ischaemia which in migraine may possibly cause subsequent prostacyclin formation and release, and therefore vasodilatation.

At a later stage in migraine, it has been suggested that head pain arises in part because of the formation of pain-producing chemicals, including eicosanoids, around distended scalp vessels. At this stage aspirin and other non-steroidal anti-inflammatory agents (NSAIDs) may act by blocking eicosanoid production locally. In this role these drugs seem to have only modest clinical effectiveness.

In the present state of knowledge there seems no biochemical basis for aspirin to act on the postulated central nervous system neurotransmitter alterations that have been suggested as possibly mediating migraine. So far, there seems no evidence at all that central nervous system eicosanoids are involved in the mechanism of the disorder.

Thus, as is the case for ergotamine, the likely mechanism of action of aspirin in migraine seems to fit better into a platelet – vascular type hypothesis of migraine pathogenesis than into those hypotheses that put the main emphasis on central neurotransmission alterations.

7.1.3 Oxygen

There are now reports that a few minutes inhalation of pure oxygen can cut short individual attacks of migrainous neuralgia (cluster headache)[37]. However, little seems to have been published on the use of oxygen in migraine. Raising the pO_2 of circulating blood has a powerful vasoconstrictor effect on the cranial circulation. Otherwise raising the pO_2 has no well-established biochemical effect in man, though it may inhibit prostacyclin synthesis[38].

It seems likely that raising the circulating pO_2 relieves the pain of cluster headache by causing vasoconstriction. This in turn suggests that the pain of this disorder is mediated by local vasodilatation, and that the vasodilatation itself produces pain. And if cranial vasodilatation causes pain in cluster headache, why should vasodilatation not also cause pain in migraine?

Another possibility, relevant to neurogenic hypotheses of migraine mechanisms, is that the oxygen therapy relieves pain in cluster headache by causing cerebral vasoconstriction which, by producing ischaemia, inactivates an essential cerebral component of the cluster headache pain-producing mechanism. However, if this were the case, the line of argument would run completely contrary to that adduced to explain pain in migraine, where it has been postulated that brain stem ischaemia causes brain stem serotonin depletion, and that this facilitates pain impulse transmission.

Thus the relatively uncomplicated pharmacological action of a high partial pressure of oxygen does provide some further evidence in favour of the vascular type hypothesis of pain production in migraine, and in cluster headache.

7.2 SUBSTANCES USED TO PREVENT MIGRAINE

A number of substances are currently employed to prevent migraine attacks. These substances vary in efficacy, and probably in mode of action. In many ways methysergide stands as the yardstick against which other migraine preventives are judged. Historically, it was one of the earliest of the currently-available agents to be employed for migraine prophylaxis, and yet to have its efficacy established by reasonably adequate controlled trials. Methysergide is customarily classified as an anti-serotonin agent. Other antiserotonin agents (which also happen to be antihistaminic agents) are also used to prevent migraine, for instance pizotifen, cyproheptadine and methdilazine, as is the β-adrenoceptor blocker propranolol, the antidepressant amitriptyline and, in particular varieties of migraine, the anticonvulsant phenytoin. As mentioned in the foregoing Section 7.1, ergotamine and aspirin have sometimes been used as migraine preventatives.

In cluster headache, as well as some of the drugs listed immediately above, lithium and synthetic adrenal glucocorticoids appear to have protective value against attacks.

7.2.1 Methysergide

The structure of the molecule resembles that of the lysergic acid moiety of ergotamine.

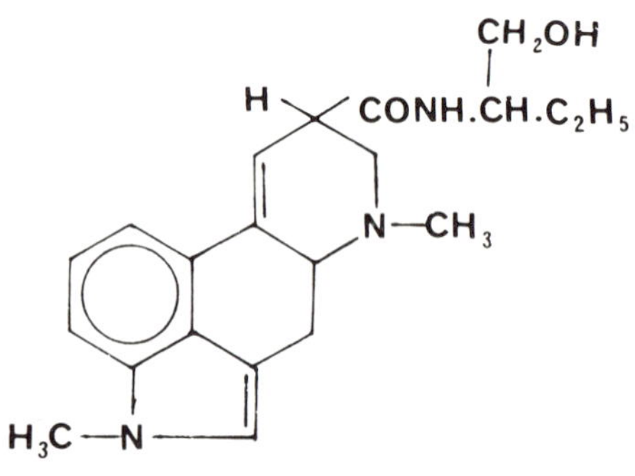

methysergide

7.2.1.1 *Clinical efficacy*

Methysergide has been used as a migraine preventative for some 25 years. Its efficacy in this role has been established in several controlled trials of adequate experimental design. There is a widespread impression that methysergide is the most effective of the currently available migraine preventives. Though also helpful in preventing cluster headache, it does not appear as effective as ergotamine in this particular role.

Despite its effectiveness, in many quarters methysergide is probably not without question the drug of first choice for migraine prophylaxis. This is so because methysergide has a number of unwanted effects, some quite serious. Thus the drug may cause nausea, hypotension or hypertension, vasospastic phenomena, a degree of alopecia, and periureteric, pleural, peritoneal and cardiac valvular fibrosis.

Methysergide has occasionally been used with some benefit in certain uncommon central nervous system disorders such as progressive supranuclear palsy, or varieties of myoclonus.

We have not traced any clinical pharmacokinetic studies of the drug. Therefore there is no knowledge that its current mode of use in clinical practice is, from the pharmacokinetic viewpoint, the most efficient possible.

7.2.1.2 *Action at a physiological level*

Many of the effects of methysergide are, from the clinical standpoint, unwanted ones – for example nausea and vomiting, hypotension or, less often, hypertension and peripheral vasoconstriction. A single dose of the drug will reduce cerebral cortical blood flow in migraineurs though not in persons with cluster headache or other types of headache; however chronic (3 – 12 weeks) therapy with the drug increases cortical blood flow in migraine sufferers[38].

Methysergide is said to potentiate analgesia produced by both endogenous and exogenous opiate agonists[39]. It will impair platelet aggregation induced by serotonin[40].

7.2.1.3 *Action at a biochemical level*

Methysergide has often been considered the paradigm of a serotonin antagonist, except in relation to the carotid vascular bed. However, since the advent of the more specific $5HT_2$ receptor antagonist ketanserin it has become obvious that methysergide, although its action appears almost entirely restricted to serotonin receptors, is a mixed agonist and antagonist. Hardebo *et al.*[41] suggested that the agonist effect occurred at lower concentrations, the antagonist at higher. The binding of methysergide to serotonin receptors may deny serotonin access to these receptors, so that in this regard the drug acts as a serotonin antagonist. Yet its binding to serotonin receptors may activate the receptors to set in train events similar to those produced by serotonin binding at the receptors. Hence it is also a serotonin agonist. Depending on which of these actions preponderates, methysergide may raise or lower blood pressure: preponderance of the agonist action could explain methysergide-induced vasospasm. According to Haigler[42] the drug does not block the action of serotonin at brain $5HT_1$ and $5HT_2$ receptors, but acts as an agonist at these receptors, and also at vascular serotonin receptors.

Methysergide will occupy serotonin uptake sites on platelets[12]. Horowski[17] stated that methysergide also has a central dopamine agonist effect, but this does not appear clinically important.

7.2.1.4 Relation of drug action to the mechanism of migraine

Methysergide prevents migraine, and for practical purposes methysergide appears to act only at serotonin receptors. Therefore one may suspect that serotonin has some relation to migraine. There is little firm evidence to take the argument beyond this point. Methysergide could be acting either in the brain, or in the circulation, or at both levels to prevent migraine. Further it could be acting as a serotonin antagonist, or as an agonist. If it acted in the latter capacity in the central nervous system it could offset the effect of the postulated fall in neurotransmitter serotonin levels that certain neurally-centered hypotheses see as important in the production of migraine. On the other hand, if the antagonist effect preponderated, a continuing blockade of central serotonin receptors should facilitate migraine unless there was also an adaptive up-regulation of receptors. Such a phenomenon is known to occur in relation to other types of central nervous system receptor[43].

If methysergide acted as a serotonin antagonist at the level of the circulation it might have a platelet anti-aggregatory effect by blocking serotonin receptors on platelets[40]. If platelets in migraine attacks did release part of their serotonin content, methysergide might prevent the released amine activating vascular wall serotonin receptors to cause vasospasm. However an agonist effect of the drug on the vessel wall in the headache-free interval and during the period of postulated serotonin release might maintain enough vascular tone to minimise vasodilatory changes in migraine attacks. Thus the combined agonist – antagonist effect of the drug could be seen as stabilising vascular wall tonus.

It should be pointed out that, if the agonist mode of action suggested immediately above is valid, methysergide may help prevent migraine simply by a direct effect on serotonin receptors in blood vessel walls. If so, there may be no serotonin-related events which are involved in the production of migraine, and which need to be influenced for the drug to protect against migraine attacks.

Thus knowledge of the biochemical pharmacology of methysergide does little to clarify the mechanism of migraine. The drug acts at too many sites, and in potentially contradictory ways, for its effects to be interpreted unambiguously.

7.2.2 The anti-serotonin anti-histamines

The drugs pizotifen, cyproheptadine and methdilazine have similar molecular structures (Figure 7.1).

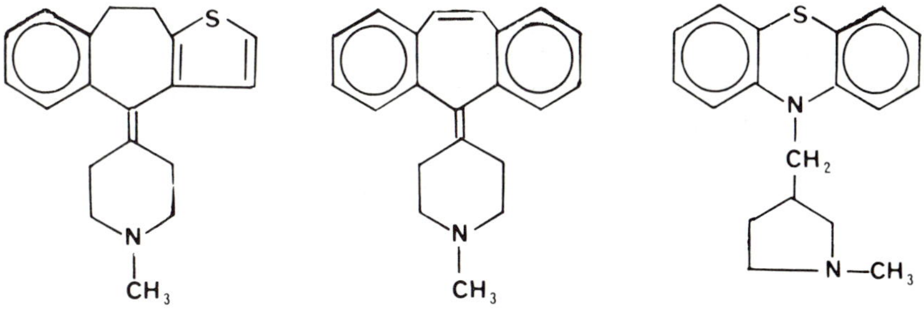

Figure 7.1 Molecular structure of pizotifen, cyproheptadine and methdilazine

7.2.2.1 Clinical efficacy

Pizotifen has been the subject of several controlled trials which have shown it more effective than placebo in preventing migraine[44]. Cyproheptadine has been subject to much less formal study in treating migraine[45], and the use of methdilazine rests on anecdotal evidence and perhaps argument from structural analogy. In practice all three drugs seem modestly effective in preventing migraine. Cyproheptadine and methdilazine have long histories of use as antihistamine and as anti-itch agents.

7.2.2.2 Action at a physiological level

All three drugs are sedatives and stimulate appetite, thus promoting weight gain. They minimise the severity of histamine-mediated allergic reactions. Some information is available about the vascular effects of pizotifen. In its own right it is a powerful constrictor of the hand veins of man, but in higher dose it also inhibits venoconstriction due to serotonin or ergotamine[4,13]. A single dose of cyproheptadine increases, but chronic intake of cyproheptadine decreases, cerebral cortical blood flow in migraineurs[30].

Pizotifen is said to have some antidepressant properties. When used chronically in migraineurs, it decreases platelet aggregability[46].

7.2.2.3 Actions at a biochemical level

All three drugs are serotonin antagonists, and are less potent in this role than is methysergide. They are also histamine antagonists at H_1 type histamine receptors, they have anticholinergic properties, and methdilazine and cyproheptadine are said to have anti-bradykinin actions. Cyproheptadine blocks dopamine receptors in the canine arterial wall[47] and acts as a serotonin agonist in the brain. The appetite promoting effects of these drugs is thought related to their altering hypothalamic (? serotoninergic) function, thus decreasing growth hormone secretion [48].

7.2.2.4 Relation of action to the mechanism of migraine

What was said about the relation between the mechanism of migraine and the central nervous system and vascular anti-serotonin effects of methysergide would also apply to these three drugs. Additionally, all three drugs have antihistamine effects, and while there is no evidence as yet to suggest that these effects produce benefit in migraine, the possibility that such antihistamine effects could benefit cluster headache should be raised.

In fact it has been suggested that pure H_1 receptor blocking agents without any antiserotonin action may protect against cluster headache[49]. One's experience is not in keeping with this suggestion, and more recently there have been reports that blockade of H_2 receptors (achieved with cimetidine or ranitidine) is not efficacious in preventing cluster headache[50]. Nor is simultaneous blockade of both H_1 and H_2 receptors[51].

In migraine bradykinin may possibly be involved in local perivascular pain production. It is not difficult to see how the antibradykinin effect of methdilazine or cyproheptadine might correct this particular aspect of the migraine mechanism. This might reduce the severity of pain during migraine attacks. However in the present state of knowledge of migraine mechanisms one would not expect blocking the action of bradykinin to prevent migraine attacks developing.

The effects of the three drugs here considered in preventing migraine are difficult to interpret in relation to the various suggested mechanisms of the disorder. The drugs are not 'clean' in relation to their known spectra of receptor effects; nor do they act at only one anatomical site in the body.

7.2.3 Tryptophan and 5-hydroxytryptophan

The serotonin aminoacid precursors tryptophan and 5-hydroxytryptophan have been used as migraine preventatives, though they have not been generally accepted as recognised therapies for the disorder.

L-5-hydroxytryptophan intake has been shown to prevent migraine[52] and L-tryptophan to have some protective effect[52,53] against the disorder. It should be noted that Bono *et al.*[54] showed that a 200 mg oral dose of 5-hydroxytryptophan in man did not alter plasma serotonin levels, though it did increase 5-hydroxyindoleacetic acid excretion. In a placebo-controlled investigation these workers showed that DL-5-hydroxytryptophan intake reduced the severity of migraine attacks, but did not reduce the attack frequency.

The effect of these two aminoacids in migraine prophylaxis suggests that serotonin is involved in the pathogenesis of the disorder. However, it is impossible to know whether changes in peripheral or central serotonin, or in both, produce the benefit.

7.2.4 β-Adrenoceptor blocking agents

A number of β-adrenoceptor blocking agents are marketed, some with a relative specificity for one or other subtype of β-receptor. Not all these drugs appear effective as migraine prophylactics. The best established β-blocker in relation to migraine prevention is propranolol, though there is evidence that atenolol[55] and timolol[56] are useful.

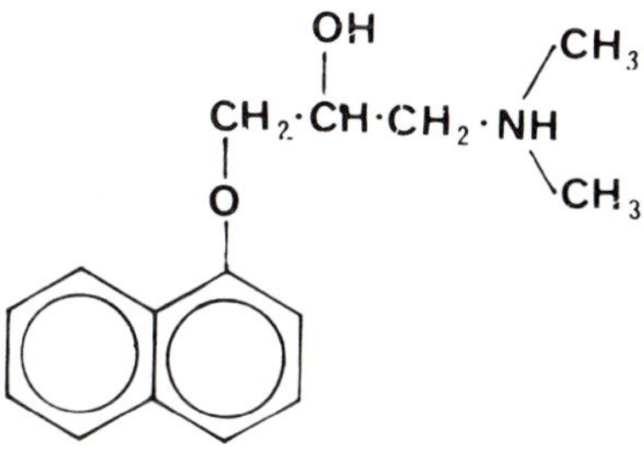

propranolol

7.2.4.1 Clinical efficacy

When propranolol came into use as an antihypertensive and anti-anginal agent clinicians began to note that the drug coincidentally appeared to reduce the frequency and severity of migraine attacks. Formal placebo- controlled trials of the drug in migraine prophylaxis were carried out[57-59]. These studies have generally shown the drug to be more effective than placebo in preventing migraine. Subsequently, similar trials have shown that atenolol and timolol are also effective, as mentioned above. However pindolol, a widely used β-blocker which possesses some intrinsic sympathomimetic activity, does not appear effective in migraine prophylaxis[60]. Nor do oxprenolol[61] or alprenolol[62], another two β-blockers with intrinsic sympathomimetic activity.

The β-blockers are useful in other roles besides that of preventing migraine. They are widely used to reduce blood pressure and prevent angina, to reduce the somatic manifestations of anxiety and thyrotoxicosis and to relieve essential tremor.

7.2.4.2 Action at a physiological level

Beta-blockers lower blood pressure by decreasing the force of myocardial contraction, and by this same mechanism may relieve angina. These drugs slow the heart (particularly those agents such as propranolol which lack intrinsic sympathomimetic activity). They tend to cause arterial and arteriolar constriction. In sufferers from migraine and cluster headache propranolol decreases cerebral blood flow[63]. Beta-blockers promote bronchial muscle and uterine contraction, and reduce the hyperglycaemic and lipolytic effects of adrenaline.

Beta-blockers act within the central nervous system to relieve essential tremor and they may alter the pattern of dreaming. They may have a local anaesthetic action. Otherwise, at ordinary dosage, they have little effect on brain function.

Propranolol increases platelet aggregability by blocking noradrenaline β-type receptors[64]. However at higher concentration (10–50 μmol/l) it inhibits the second wave of adrenaline and ADP induced aggregation and blocks platelet serotonin release[65].

7.2.4.3 Action at a biochemical level

Propranolol has conventionally been regarded as a β-adrenoceptor blocking agent, acting as an antagonist at both β_1 and β_2 receptors. The other β-blockers useful in migraine prophylaxis possess the same mode of action, and in general they lack intrinsic sympathomimetic activity.

More recently a number of lines of evidence have accumulated indicating that propranolol also affects various functions mediated by serotonin. Fozard[66] stated that the drug blocked serotonin receptors in the brain, while Green and Grahame-Smith[67], Middlemiss *et al.*[68] and Weinstock *et al.*[69] stated that it inhibited central serotoninergic neurotransmission.

Propranolol does not appear to interfere with eicosanoid synthesis by cerebral vessels[18].

7.2.4.4 Relation of drug action to the mechanism of migraine

The discovery of the effect of propranolol on serotonin mechanisms has in some ways confounded the interpretation of the drug's role *vis à vis* the mechanism of migraine. If the drug were seen purely in a β-adrenoceptor blocking role this mechanism of action could appear to correlate with (a) blockade of the noradrenergic discharges from the locus coeruleus that Lance[70] suggested might alter pial vascular reactivity in migraine, or with (b) blockade of the postulated sympathetic overactivity that occurs in migraine, possibly preventing the presence of excess circulating noradrenaline and thus avoiding a circumstance which may initiate the sequence of free fatty acid release causing platelet activation which causes subsequent elements of the migraine mechanism[71,72]. If propranolol acted as a β-blocker, the effectiveness of the drug in migraine prevention could then be seen as supporting either one variant of the neural type hypothesis of migraine mechanism, or, perhaps a little remotely, one variant of the platelet–vascular type of hypothesis, in which neural events instigated the intravascular changes.

However, more possibilities than these exist. It is also possible that the migraine-preventing actions of propranolol may involve both central nervous system and platelet serotonin-mediated effects. The known biochemical actions of propranolol have the potential for interfering at so many points in different suggested migraine mechanisms that the effectiveness of the drug in migraine prevention provides no particularly strong evidence in favour of one mechanism over another.

7.2.5 Amitriptyline

Amitriptyline is a widely used tricyclic antidepressant which forms a biologically-active *N*-desmethylated metabolite, nortriptyline.

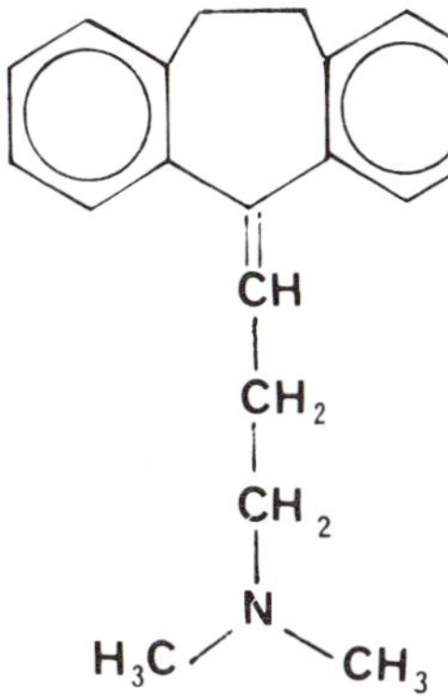

amitriptyline

7.2.5.1 Clinical efficacy

Placebo-controlled studies have shown that amitriptyline, generally in the dose range 50–75 mg daily, is a reasonably effective migraine prophylactic agent[73,74]. The drug's main use in medicine is in treating endogenous (primary) depression. Some studies have suggested that it is useful in treating contraction headache[75]. However it is possible that there was underlying migraine in some of the instances of contraction headache investigated. Therefore benefit that accrued from the antimigraine actions of amitriptyline may have been attributed to an effect on contraction headache.

7.2.5.2 Action at a physiological level

Amitriptyline has no mood altering effect in non-depressed persons. However it has sedative and anticholinergic actions (dry mouth, blurred vision, tendency to urine retention and constipation), may cause hypotension and, in overdosage, can cause disturbance of cardiac rhythm, confusion and convulsions.

7.2.5.3 Action at a biochemical level

Amitryptiline has a number of mechanisms of action on the nervous system[76]. It is a centrally and peripherally-acting anticholinergic agent at muscarinic type acetylcholine receptors. It blocks serotonin reuptake after discharge of this amine neurotransmitter from axon terminals. The amitriptyline metabolite nortriptyline blocks noradrenaline reuptake into nerve terminals. Thus amitriptyline increases both catecholamine and indolealkylamine concentrations in synaptic clefts. Fozard[66] stated that amitriptyline blocks serotonin receptors. It is known that imipramine, a drug structurally related to amitriptyline, acts on platelets to block serotonin uptake[67], and it seems possible that amitriptyline has a similar action. Platelets cannot synthesise serotonin[78]. Therefore unless serotonin uptake and reuptake mechanisms in platelets are different, platelets could become serotonin depleted from the effects of amitriptyline. They would then have little or no serotonin to release.

7.2.5.4 Relation of drug action to the mechanism of migraine

The known biochemical pharmacology of amitriptyline would explain how the drug might enhance central noradrenergic neurotransmission. Whether this would benefit migraine is problematical, even accepting that there may be altered central noradrenergic neurotransmission in the disorder. Propranolol, which interferes with central noradrenergic neurotransmission, a contrary action to that of amitriptyline, also prevents migraine. Amitriptyline might cause increased synaptic serotonin concentrations in the substantia gelatinosa. This might impair rostral conduction of pain impulses and thus reduce the pain of migraine. Such an action, which might apply in a number of forms of somatic pain apart from migraine, could reduce the severity of migraine attacks regardless of whether or not there was an impairment of brain stem serotonin functioning in the disorder. It is a moot point whether the antidepressant action of amitriptyline, mediated by altered central noradrenergic or serotoninergic neurotransmission, or by some other mechanism, could influence migraine.

The action of amitriptyline could alter platelet function by depleting platelets of serotonin. Thus certain factors which appear to instigate migraine by promoting serotonin release from platelets would no longer be able to achieve this effect.

Amitriptyline has too many actions, in the central nervous system and more peripherally, for its effectiveness in migraine prophylaxis to throw much light on the mechanisms of the disorder.

7.2.6 Monoamine oxidase inhibitors

A number of monoamine oxidase inhibitors are available but only one, phenelzine, appears to have been shown useful in migraine prophylaxis.

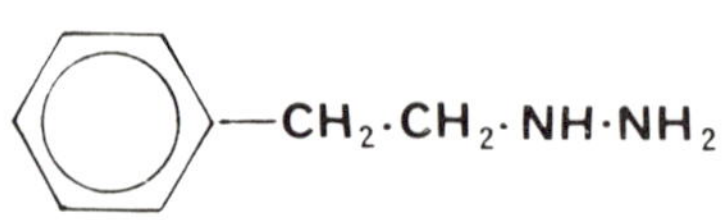

phenelzine

7.2.6.1 Clinical efficacy

There are at least two reports of uncontrolled studies[79,80] showing that phenelzine is effective in preventing migraine. The drug does not appear to have come into widespread use for this purpose, however. This may be due to the well known hazards of using this type of drug, and the consequent dietary restriction that must be imposed on patients.

Monoamine oxidase inhibitors (MAOIs) are used mainly in psychiatry, to treat certain varieties of otherwise refactory depression, and for obsessive–compulsive states.

7.2.6.2 Action at the physiological level

Monoamine oxidase inhibitors have no mood-elevating effects in mentally-normal persons. If taken in the absence of dietary sources of amines, these drugs have little effect in normal persons, though they tend to lower blood pressure.

7.2.6.3 Action at the biochemical level

Phenelzine inhibits monoamine oxidase of both type A and type B. The drug therefore diminishes the degradation of both catecholamines (dopamine, noradrenaline and adrenaline) and serotonin in the nervous system and in peripheral tissues.

7.2.6.4 Relation of drug action to the mechanism of migraine

One has reservations about how well founded is the efficacy of phenelzine in migraine prophylaxis. Accepting that the drug is effective, the benefit could be explained in terms of neural hypotheses of migraine production which invoke impairment of central serotoninergic or noradrenergic activity (phenelzine would then be acting much as amitriptyline might act – Section 7.2.4 – though through a different molecular mechanism). However phenelzine might also act in migraine by increasing circulating biogenic amine levels, since it would cause decreased degradation of the amines. It seems fruitless to try to relate the action of phenelzine to the (now somewhat uncertain) diminution in platelet monoamine oxidase type B reported as occurring during migraine.

Basically, the molecular alterations due to monoamine oxidase inhibition appear to involve too many substances at too many sites in the body to throw much light on the mechanism of migraine.

7.2.7 Flunarazine

Flunarazine is a comparatively recently introduced calcium antagonist whose pharmacology and pattern of use are not yet fully worked out.

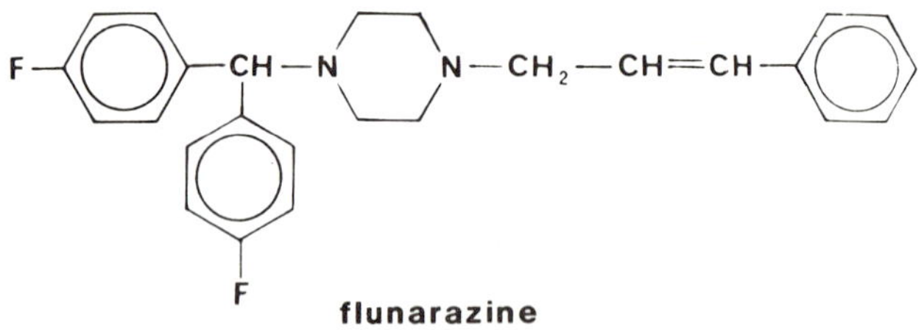

flunarazine

7.2.7.1 Clinical efficacy

There are now several placebo-controlled trials demonstrating that intake of flunarazine confers protection against migraine (decrease in the frequency rather than in the severity of attacks)[81-83]. The drug's main contemporary use appears to be in preventing angina. Other calcium channel blocking agents,such as nimodipine[84,85] and verapamil[86], are reported to prevent migraine. Cyproheptadine and amitriptyline, each of which is discussed elsewhere in this chapter as a migraine prophylactic, are now known to have calcium channel blocking actions[87].

7.2.7.2 Action at a physiological level

Flunarazine appears to relax contracted smooth muscle (vascular and bronchial). It improves brain tolerance to oxygen deprivation in experimental animals and has vestibular depressant and anticonvulsant actions in animals and man[88].

7.2.7.3 Action at a biochemical level

Flunarazine seems to impair smooth muscle contraction by blocking Ca^{2+} channels in cell membranes, thus preventing the Ca^{2+} influx that is a preliminary to shortening of actomyosin chains in muscle. It may interfere with Ca^{2+} mediated serotonin release from platelets.

7.2.7.4 Relation of drug action to mechanism of migraine

Although an action within the central nervous system cannot be excluded, the effect of flunarazine in decreasing migraine could be explained by an impaired ability of cranial arteries to go into spasm during migraine attacks. Thus, in the present state of knowledge, the effectiveness of flunarazine in migraine prevention could be seen as supporting the view that vascular spasm played a role in the pathogenesis of the disorder.

7.2.8 Phenytoin

Phenytoin is a widely used anticonvulsant, but there is some anecdotal evidence of efficacy in certain uncommon varieties of migraine.

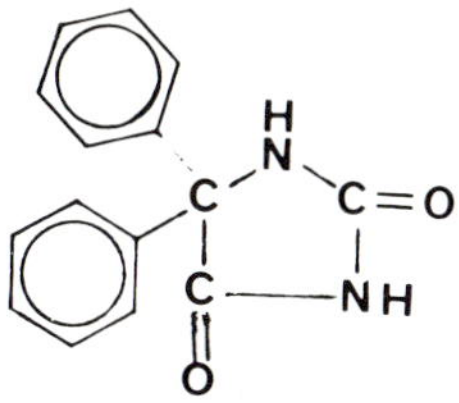

phenytoin

7.2.8.1 Clinical efficacy

It is a matter of clinical observation that phenytoin is occasionally a very effective preventive for certain patterns of adult migraine, particularly for attacks in which the aura comprises unilateral somatic sensory changes or dysphasia, and for so-called basilar artery migraine[89]. Phenytoin also seems of some use in preventing childhood migraine, but does not appear to be effective in preventing adult common migraine or classical migraine with a visual aura.

The main use of phenytoin in medicine is as an anticonvulsant. The drug is occasionally employed to treat myotonia and certain cardiac arrhythmias.

7.2.8.2 Action at a physiological level

Phenytoin acts by inhibiting the spread of epileptic activity, rather than by preventing the initiation of such activity[90]. Considerable detail as to its effects on electrical function of the nervous system is available elsewhere[91]. There does not seem to have been any detailed study of vascular effects of the drug.

7.2.8.3 Action at a molecular level

Phenytoin has a number of known biochemical effects[90,91], including activation of the enzyme Na^+, K^+ linked adenosine triphosphatase, and impairment of Na^+ conductance through cell membranes. Its essential mechanism of action, even in epilepsy, is not yet certain.

7.2.8.4 Relation of drug action to the mechanism of migraine

The prophylactic effect of phenytoin applies only in certain clinical varieties of migraine, and not to migraine in general. Phenytoin is known to act on skeletal muscle (in myotonia), and on the myocardium as well as on the nervous system. Therefore the action of the drug in preventing certain varieties of migraine need not necessarily occur at central nervous system level. Perhaps the inference to be drawn from the effectiveness of phenytoin in certain types of migraine is that the alteration of function in certain brain areas during these types of migraine, or in the blood vessels supplying these areas, may not be biochemically identical with that which occurs in the brain or its vessels in other more common varieties of migraine. Probably no conclusion about any general mechanisms of migraine pathogenesis can be drawn from the mode of action of a drug with so limited a spectrum of efficacy in the disorder.

7.2.9 Adrenal glucocorticoids

Although adrenal corticosteroids have no established role in migraine, except perhaps for controlling the rare status migrainicus, prednisone has been used with success in suppressing cluster headache when lesser remedies have failed. It is believed that prednisone acts pharmacologically only after it undergoes biological oxidation at the 11 position to form prednisolone.

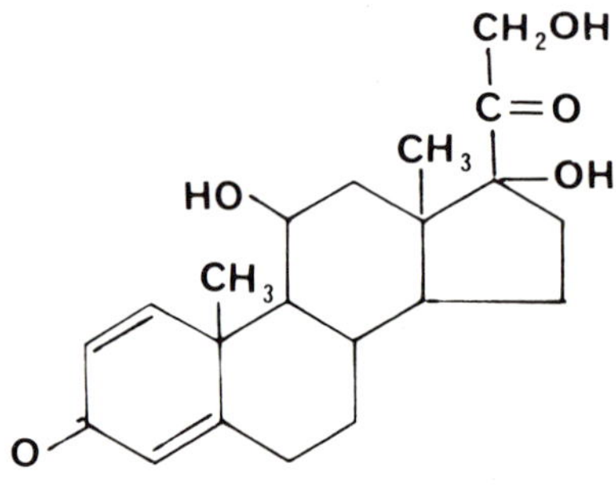

prednisolone

7.2.9.1 Clinical efficacy

There are publications attesting to the efficacy of prednisone in terminating bouts of cluster headache[92,93].

In contemporary therapeutics prednisone and related glucocorticoids are used for a variety of indications, benefit for which involves the anti-inflammatory, oedema-reducing, antineoplastic and hormonal replacement effects of the steroid.

7.2.9.2 Action at a physiological level

Glucocorticoids decrease vascular permeability, accelerate the destruction of certain types of cell, raise blood pressure by causing Na^+, Cl^- and water retention, and cause protein breakdown and hyperglycaemia.

7.2.9.3 Action at a biochemical level

Glucocorticoids act at specific cellular steroid receptors where they mimic the action of the natural adrenal steroid cortisol (hydrocortisone). However, glucocorticoids have relatively less Na^+, Cl^- and water-retaining potency than the natural steroid.

7.2.9.4 Relation of drug action to the mechanism of headache

The known mechanisms of steroid action do not provide any obvious basis for the effectiveness of these drugs in preventing attacks of cluster headache. One could conceive that an anti-inflammatory action might mitigate the severity of individual cluster attacks, but it is difficult to see how such a mechanism could have a preventive role. There might be some basis for arguing that the steroid action in cluster headache would be more likely to occur at a vascular than a neural level. The effectiveness of glucocorticoids in the prophylaxis of cluster headache throws no light on the mechanisms of migraine.

7.2.10 Lithium

Oral lithium carbonate therapy is reputedly of use in controlling chronic cluster headache[94].

7.2.10.1 Clinical efficacy

There are a number of published studies which indicate that continued lithium therapy may slowly bring chronic cluster headache under control[94] and may prevent relapse if given in the attack free period between clusters. Interestingly, lithium is reputed to make migraine worse[95].

The major use of lithium in medicine is in controlling mania, and in preventing relapses of manic-depressive psychosis.

7.2.10.2 Action at a physiological level

Lithium does not appear to have any appreciable mood depressing effect in persons whose mood is normal. It may stabilise mood in persons prone to endogenous depression. In high dosage the drug causes tremor and mental changes.

Continued lithium therapy in patients with cluster headache does not alter cerebral blood flow measured with the ^{133}Xe technique, nor cerebral vascular reactivity to change in pCO_2 or pO_2[96].

7.2.10.3 Action at a biochemical level

The body handles Li^+ as it handles Na^+. The cation is excreted via the kidneys. Lithium appears to enhance the turnover of biogenic amines in the nervous system so that reduced amounts of neurotransmitter are stored in axon terminals. Consequently there is decreased release of noradrenaline and serotonin into synaptic clefts in response to neuronal activity. Thus functionally lithium impairs monoaminergic neurotransmission.

7.2.10.4 Relation of drug action to mechanism of headache

The mechanism whereby lithium brings chronic cluster headache under control remains obscure. The role of the ion in preventing cluster headache seems to offer no help in understanding the mechanisms involved in migraine.

7.3 CHEMICALS WHICH PROVOKE HEADACHES

A number of drugs are known to be capable of provoking attacks of migraine, or of cluster headache. Certain of these agents are sometimes used as experimental tools for that purpose.

7.3.1 Reserpine

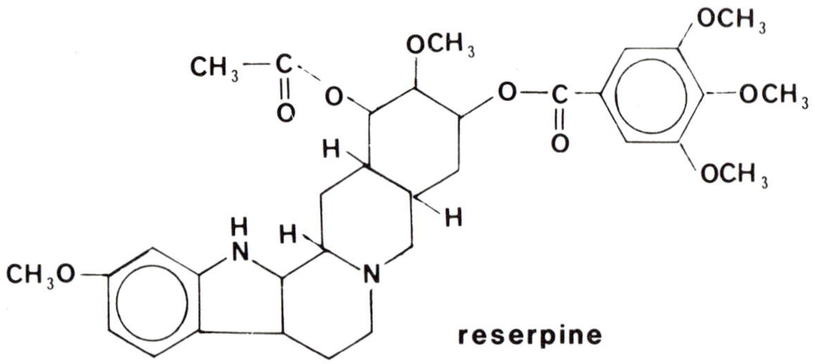

reserpine

7.3.1.1 Efficacy

When reserpine came into use as an antihypertensive agent more than a quarter of a century ago, its side-effects were found to include nasal stuffiness, depression and headache. It became recognised that the drug could provoke migraine in those predisposed to this disorder. The drug has since been used in some experimental studies to induce migraine attacks[97,98].

7.3.1.2 Action at a physiological level

Reserpine lowers blood pressure by decreasing peripheral resistance. It causes nasal stuffiness because of the local nasal vasodilatation produced. Its mood-altering effect arises centrally.

7.3.1.3 Action at a biochemical level

Reserpine causes the release of stored biogenic amines from nerve terminals in the central and peripheral sympathetic nervous systems, and from storage granules in platelets. The resulting deficiency in stored amines causes reduced amine concentrations at post-synaptic receptors after neural activity. After a reserpine injection there is a reduced serotonin content of platelets which persists for 4–6 weeks[98], and increased urinary excretion of 5-hydroxyindoleacetic acid and vanillylmandelic acid[97].

7.3.1.4 Relation of action to mechanism of migraine

Administration of reserpine to predisposed persons is soon followed by migraine attacks, though with intake of the drug over several weeks the tendency to activation of migraine disappears[98]. In fact, a double blind study[99] showed that reserpine, given every second or third day, had a migraine-preventing effect. In terms of the platelet–vascular type of hypothesis of migraine pathogenesis reserpine might be seen as provoking platelet serotonin release which thus instigates the migraine mechanism. With continuing exposure to reserpine platelets become so depleted of serotonin that further doses of the drug can no longer release much of the amine from platelets. Therefore the activation of migraine does not persist indefinitely if reserpine intake is continued.

Reserpine intake would be expected to produce an initial efflux of dopamine, noradrenaline, adrenaline and serotonin into the relevant synapses of the nervous system. Yet this event often seems to be followed by an attack of migraine. This is contrary to what would be expected from the neural hypotheses of migraine pathogenesis which relate attacks of the disorder to serotonin depletion, rather than temporary excess of the amine, in certain pathways in the brain stem. Further, with continued reserpine therapy, which would ultimately cause reduced serotonin release into synapses, there would exist the set of circumstances invoked in the neural hypotheses of migraine pathogenesis. Yet in these circumstances the tendency to induced migraine attacks seems to lessen, not increase. Of course, in such circumstances the expected consequences of persisting serotonin deficiency at central synapses may be to some extent offset by a postulated 'up-regulation' of post-synaptic serotonin receptors.

In all, the known mode of action of reserpine, taken in conjunction with the time pattern of its capacity to induce migraine, appears more in favour of the platelet–vascular hypotheses of migraine pathogenesis than current versions of the neurally-centred hypotheses.

7.3.2 Glyceryl trinitrate (nitroglycerine)

$$\begin{array}{l} CH_2.O.NO_2 \\ | \\ CH.O.NO_2 \\ | \\ CH_2.O.NO_2 \end{array}$$

glyceryl trinitrate

7.3.2.1 Clinical efficacy

Glyceryl trinitrate, when used to relieve anginal pain, sometimes produces brief but fairly severe throbbing headache. Less often, the drug appears capable of activating migraine[100], even when applied locally to the scalp[101]. Nitroglycerine may also cause attacks of cluster headache during periods of activity of the disorder. However, it is salutary to remember that, in the past, glyceryl trinitrate was a component of Gowers' mixture which was widely used as a migraine preventative.

7.3.2.2 Action at a physiological level

Glyceryl trinitrate is a potent short-acting vasodilator. The drug relaxes smooth muscle at most sites in the body. In monkeys it dilates both intracranial and extracranial arteries[102].

7.3.2.3 Action at a biochemical level

The mechanism of action of glyceryl trinitrate at a molecular level is uncertain.

7.3.2.4 Relation of drug action to mechanisms of migraine

As far as is known the effects of glyceryl trinitrate are purely on the vascular system. There is no known action on the central nervous system. Therefore the effect of glyceryl trinitrate in activating migraine correlates better with vascular than with neural hypotheses of migraine pathogenesis.

7.3.3 Caffeine

Caffeine, a methylxanthine, is present in beverages such as coffee and tea, and is a component of a number of proprietary analgesic preparations.

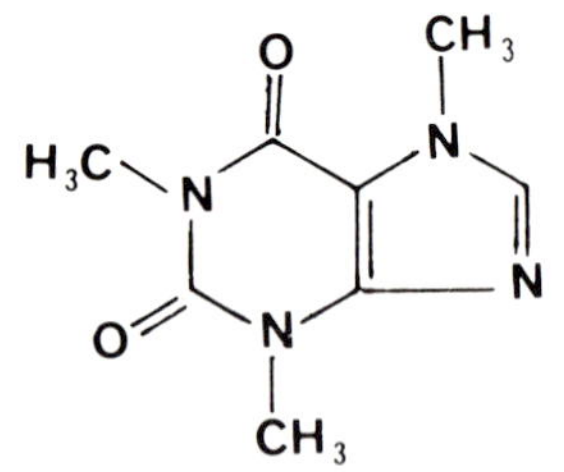

caffeine

7.3.3.1 Clinical efficacy

Caffeine has a popular reputation for relieving milder migraine. This reputation appears to derive in part from the alleged effects of coffee in these circumstances, it being assumed that caffeine is the active ingredient responsible for the benefit. Caffeine may be capable of enhancing the absorption of orally administered ergotamine[103]. There are reports that frequent intake of caffeine can cause rebound migraine-like headache, which is relieved by further caffeine intake[104,105],thus promoting a vicious circle.

7.3.3.2 Action at a physiological level

Caffeine is a mild cerebral and cardiac stimulant, a bronchodilator and a diuretic. In overdosage it can causes a tendency to cardiac arrhythmia. It dilates peripheral blood vessels, but constricts the cerebral circulation. Caffeine increases gastric secretion of acid and pepsin.

7.3.3.3 Action at a biochemical level

Caffeine inhibits the enzyme cyclic nucleotide phosphodiesterase and thus delays the breakdown of cyclic adenosine monophosphate. It is often considered that the effects of caffeine are mediated through the increased cAMP levels so produced. Caffeine may also inhibit the effects of adenosine.

7.3.3.4 Relation of drug action to mechanism of migraine

Caffeine has direct effects on both the central nervous system and vascular smooth muscle, and details of its effects on the neural pathways involved in migraine have not yet been worked out. Therefore it is difficult to argue from the effects of caffeine on migraine to the mechanisms of the disorder.

7.3.4 Ergotamine

There are a number of published assertions that too frequent an intake of ergotamine in migraine can cause rebound headache requiring further ergotamine for its relief[106-108]. Perusal of these reports shows that, in many instances, the ergotamine appears to have been administered in preparations also containing caffeine, and the role of caffeine withdrawal in provoking migraine has been mentioned above (Section 7.3.3). When used for cluster headache, ergotamine itself can be injected two or three times a day for several days without such rebound headache occurring. One therefore wonders if at least some instances of so-called ergotamine withdrawal headache may really be caffeine-withdrawal headache.

7.3.5 Histamine

Histamine has already been considered (Section 3.4) as a possible factor in the pathogenesis of migraine and it will be considered again in relation to cluster headache (Chapter 10). Histamine is mentioned in the present section only in its role as a headache precipitating agent. Histamine does not appear to provoke migraine with any frequency. However during clusters, though not between clusters, histamine is capable of triggering individual attacks of cluster headache. This phenomenon has been known since the work of Horton[109], who on the basis of the finding termed the syndrome 'histaminic cephalalgia'.

7.3.6 Zimelidine

Zimelidine is an antidepressant drug that began to come into use in clinical medicine, but was withdrawn because of occasional but serious neurotoxic effects.

It, and its *N*-desalkyl derivative, which is a biotransformation product in man, are believed to act by impeding serotonin reuptake into nerve terminals and serotonin uptake into platelets.

The use of zimelidine has been reported to increase the frequency and severity of migraine attacks[66]. Such an effect would not be expected if the neural type

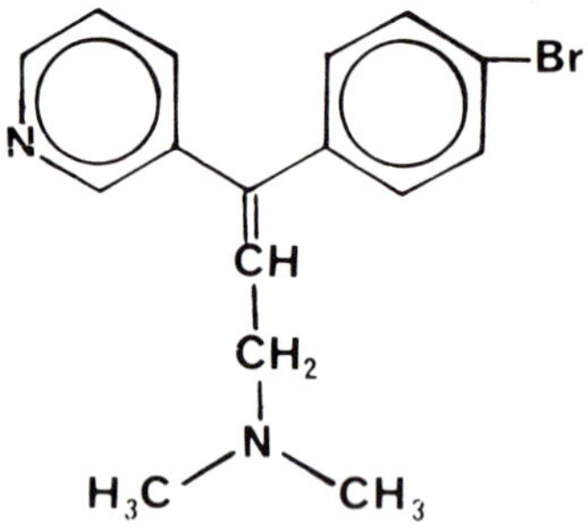

zimelidine

of hypothesis of migraine mechanism applied. Zimelidine should reverse, not worsen, the postulated depletion of neurotransmitter serotonin that, in terms of this hypothesis, causes migraine. However, if zimelidine decreased platelet serotonin uptake and raised serotonin concentrations in plasma water, the events implicit in the platelet – vascular type of hypothesis of the migraine mechanism would have occurred.

7.3.7 Ethyl alcohol

In some migraineurs many different varieties of beverage containing ethyl alcohol appear non-specifically capable of producing attacks of migraine. In other migraine sufferers only particular beverages, commonly red wines, appear to possess this capacity. In still other migraineurs ethyl alcohol intake never seems to cause attacks of migraine. By way of contrast, in persons with cluster headache the intake of any form of alcohol is commonly followed within 2 or 3 hours by an attack, but this occurs only while a cluster is present. In the interval between clusters, alcohol intake does not produce attacks.

The difficulty in interpreting these observations is that alcohol-containing beverages contain not only ethyl alcohol but trace amounts of a variety of substances including amines, which differ from beverage to beverage and which may not always have been completely categorised chemically. It is therefore impossible to know whether the alcohol itself, or some other constituent of the beverages, provokes the headaches. Consequently one cannot argue from a known provoking agent to the biochemical mechanism of migraine or of cluster headache.

7.3.8 Foodstuffs

While a considerable variety of foodstuffs may provoke migraine attacks in particular individuals[110,111] the exact chemical constituents responsible have rarely been identified. In a careful study Egger *et al.*[112] obtained evidence that migraine attacks in a group of children were related to exposure to several foods rather than to a single food. Merrett *et al.*[113] failed to detect the increased incidence of specific IgE and IgG_4 that would be expected if such dietary migraine were mediated through allergic mechanisms. Therefore one cannot deduce much about the mechanism of production of migraine from the chemical nature of the provoking agents in foods.

7.3.9 Sodium chloride

The evidence that a NaCl load may precipitate migraine[114] was considered in Section 6.1.1

7.4 INFERENCES ABOUT THE MECHANISM OF MIGRAINE AND CLUSTER HEADACHE

Drawing inferences about pathogenesis from the actions of drugs and chemicals on a disease often proves a somewhat uncertain affair. The inferences depend very heavily on knowledge of the modes of action of the drugs and chemicals in question, but these substances may have other pertinent, as yet unknown, actions. With this reservation, when the known modes of actions of the chemicals discussed in this chapter are related to the types of hypothesis of migraine pathogenesis that are in currency, virtually none of the evidence appears unambiguously in favour of the various types of neural hypothesis of migraine pathogenesis. Some of the evidence is consistent with the neural type of hypothesis. However a few items, such as the effects of reserpine, are difficult to reconcile with this type of neural hypothesis. On the other hand no item of evidence considered in the present chapter is irreconcilable with the platelet – vascular line of hypothesis. Almost every item of evidence is consistent with this line of hypothesis, and several items, e.g. the effects of ergotamine, aspirin, oxygen and nitroglycerine, are clearly in favour of the circulation-centered hypothesis.

Overall, one would have to conclude that the inferences that can be drawn from the known modes of action of the various exogenous chemical substances that influence migraine tend to favour the view that the phenomena of migraine arise from altered platelet and vascular behaviour.

References

1. Berde, B. and Schild, H.O. (eds.) (1978). *Ergot Alkaloids and Related Compounds.* Berlin: Springer
2. Eadie, M.J. (1983). Ergotamine pharmacokinetics in man: an editorial. *Cephalalgia,* **3,** 135–138
3. Saxena, P.R. (1974). Selective carotid vasoconstriction by ergotamine as a relevant mechanism in its antimigraine effect. *Archives de Neurobiologica,* **37,** 301–315
4. Aellig, W.H. (1982). Agonists and antagonists of 5- hydroxytryptamine on venomotor receptors. *Advances in Neurology,* **33,** 321–324
5. Spierings, E.L.H. and Saxena, P.R. (1980). Antimigraine drugs and cranial arteriovenous shunting in the cat. *Neurology,* **30,** 696–701
6. Spierings, E.L.H. and Saxena, P.R. (1980). The action of ergotamine on the distribution of carotid blood flow – the migraine shunt theory revisited. *Headache,* **20,** 143–145
7. Spierings, E.L.H. and Saxena, P.R. (1982). Pharmacology of arteriovenous anastomoses. *Advances in Neurology,* **33,** 291–294
8. Raskin, N.H. (1981). Pharmacology of migraine. *Annual Review of Pharmacology,* **21,** 463–478
9. Norris, J.W., Hachinski, V.C. and Cooper, P.W. (1975). Changes in cerebral blood flow during a migraine attack. *British Medical Journal,* **3,** 676–684
10. Hachinski, V., Norris, J.W., Edmeads, J. and Cooper, P.W. (1978). Ergotamine and cerebral blood flow. *Stroke,* **9,** 594–596
11. Hachinski, V.C., Norris, J.W., Cooper, P.W. and Edmeads, J.G. (1978). Migraine and the cerebral circulation. In Greene, R. (ed.). *Current Concepts in Migraine Research.* New York: Raven Press, 11–15
12. Hilton, B.P. and Zilkha, K.J. (1974). Effects of ergotamine and methysergide on blood platelet aggregation responses in migrainous subjects. *Journal of Neurology, Neurosurgery and Psychiatry,* **37,** 593–597
13. Aellig, W.H. (1978). Clinical-pharmacological experiments with pizotifin (Sanomigran^{R}) on superficial hand veins of man. In Greene, R. (ed.) *Current Concepts in Migraine Research.* New York: Raven Press, 53–62
14. Müller-Schweinitzer, E. (1978). Studies on the 5-HT receptor in vascular smooth muscle. *Research and Clinical Studies in Headache,* **6,** 6–12
15. Müller-Schweinitzer, E. and Fanchamps, A. (1982). Effects on arterial receptors of ergot derivatives used in migraine. *Advances in Neurology,* **33,** 343–356
16. Fozard, J.R. (1975). The animal pharmacology of drugs in the treatment of migraine. In Saxena, P.R. (ed.) *Migraine and Related Headaches.* Uden: Sandoz, 93–118
17. Horowski, R. (1982). Some aspects of the dopaminergic action of ergot derivatives and their role in the treatment of migraine. *Advances in Neurology,* **33,** 325–334
18. Gaudet, R.J., Maurer, P., Levine, L. and Moskowitz, M.A. (1979). Prostaglandins: accumulation in brain after transient ischemia and in vitro synthesis by cerebral microvessels. *Headache,* **19,** 245
19. Spierings, E.L.H., Zijlstra, F.J. and Vincent, J.E. (1981). Effect of ergotamine on prostaglandin synthesis. In Rose, F.C. and Zilkha, K.J. (eds.) *Progress in Migraine Research. 1.* London: Pitman, 151–155
20. Zijlstra, F.J., Spierings, E.L.H. and Vincent, J.E. (1980). The effect of ergotamine on prostaglandin formation in guinea pigs ear slices. *Headache,* **20,** 305–306
21. Zijlstra, F.J., Spierings, E.L.H. and Vincent, J.E. (1981). Effect of ergotamine on platelet prostaglandin synthesis – in vitro and in vivo experiments. *Cephalalgia,* **1,** 25–27
22. Campbell, A.W. (1933). The treatment of migraine. *Medical Journal of Australia,* **1,** 36–37
23. Matthews, W.B. (1963). *Practical Neurology.* Oxford: Blackwell Scientific Publications
24. Wilkinson, M.I.P. (1975). The treatment of migraine. In Saxena, P.R. (ed.). *Migraine and Related Headache.* Uden: Sandoz, 141–156
25. Ross-Lee, L.M., Eadie, M.J. and Tyrer, J.H. (1982). Aspirin treatment of migraine attacks: clinical observations. *Cephalalgia,* **2,** 71–76
26. O'Neill, B.P. and Mann, J.D. (1978). Aspirin prophylaxis in migraine. *Lancet,* **2,** 1179–1181
27. Masel, B.E., Chesson, A.L., Peters, B.H., Levin, H.S. and Alperin, J.B. (1980). Platelet antagonists in migraine prophylaxis. A clinical trial using aspirin and dipyridamole. *Head-*

antagonists in migraine prophylaxis. A clinical trial using aspirin and dipyridamole. *Headache,* **20,** 13–18

28. Ryan, R.E. Sr. and Ryan, R.E. Jr.(1982). The use of platelet inhibitors in migraine. *Advances in Neurology,* **33,** 247–252
29. Mikkelsen, B.M. and Falk, J.V. (1982). Prophylactic treatment of migraine with tolfenamic acid. A comparative double-blind crossover study between tolfenamic acid and placebo. *Acta Neurologica Scandinavica,* **66,** 105–111
30. Amano, T. and Meyer, J.S. (1982). Prostaglandin inhibition and cerebrovascular control in patients with headache. *Headache,* **22,** 52–59
31. Pickard, D.J., Rose, J.E., Cooke, M.B.D., Blair, I. Mc.L. and Strathdee, A. (1977). The effect of salicylate on cerebral blood flow in man. *Acta Neurologica Scandinavica,* Suppl. 64, 422–423
32. Zucker, M.B. and Peterson, J. (1968). Inhibition of adenosine diphosphate-induced secondary aggregation and other platelet functions by acetylsalicylic acid ingestion. *Proceedings of the Society for Experimental Biology,* **127,** 547–551
33. Vane, J.R. (1971). Inhibition of prostaglandin synthesis as a mechanism of action for aspirin-like drugs. *Nature New Biology,* **231,** 232–235
34. De Gaetano, G., Cerletti, C. and Bertele, V. (1982). Pharmacology of antiplatelet drugs and clinical trials on thrombosis prevention: a difficult link. *Lancet,* **2,** 974– 977
35. Merino, J., Livio, M., Rajtar, G. and DeGaetano, G.I. (1980). Salicylate reverses in vitro aspirin inhibition of rat platelet and vascular prostaglandin generation. *Biochemical Pharmacology,* **29,** 1093–1096
36. Hamberg, M. (1972). Inhibition of prostaglandin synthesis in man. *Biochemical and Biophysical Research Communications,* **49,** 720–726
37. Kudrow, L. (1981). Response of cluster headache attacks to oxygen inhalation. *Headache,* **21,** 1–4
38. Amano, T. and Meyer, J.S. (1982). Cerebrovascular changes in patients with headache during antiserotoninergic treatment. *Headache,* **22,** 249–255
39. Bartolini, A., Malmberg, P., Bartolini, R. and Giotti, A. (1982). Effect of antimigraine drugs on nonopioid analgesia. In Critchley, M., Friedman, A.P., Gorini, S. and Sicuteri, F. (eds.). *Migraine: Physiopathological and Clinical Concepts. Advances in Neurology,* **33,** 89–97
40. De Gaetano, G. and Garattini, S. (eds.) (1978). *Platelets: a Multidisciplinary Approach.* New York: Raven Press
41. Hardebo, J.E., Edvinsson, L., Owman, Ch. and Svendgaard, N- Aa. (1978). Potentiation and antagonism of serotonin effects on intracranial and extracranial vessels. Possible implications in migraine. *Neurology,* **28,** 64–70
42. Haigler, H. (1982). Characteristics of extravascular serotonin receptors in the brain. In Critchley, M., Friedman, A.P., Gorini, S. and Sicuteri, F. (eds.). *Headache – Physiopathogenesis and Clinical Concepts. Advances in Neurology,* **33,** 283–289
43. Kurlan, R. and Shoulson, I. (1982). Up and down regulation: clinical significance of nervous system receptor–drug interaction. *Clinical Neuropharmacology,* **5,** 345–350
44. Speight, T.M. and Avery, G.S. (1972). Pizotifen (BC-105): a review of its pharmacological properties and its therapeutic efficacy in vascular headaches. *Drugs,* **3,** 159–203
45. Lance, J.W., Anthony, M. and Somerville, B. (1970). Comparative trial of serotonin antagonists in the management of migraine. *British Medical Journal,* **2,** 327– 330
46. Mazal, S. and Rachmilewitz, E.A. (1980). The effect of an antiserotonin agent pizotifen on platelet aggregability in migraine patients. *Journal of Neurology, Neurosurgery and Psychiatry,* **43,** 1137–1140
47. Gilbert, J.C. and Goldberg, L.J. (1975). Characterization by cyproheptadine of the dopamine-induced contraction in canine isolated arteries. *Journal of Pharmacology and Experimental Therapeutics,* **193,** 435–442
48. Smythe, G.A. and Lazarus, L. (1974). Suppression of human growth hormone secretion by melatonin and cyproheptadine. *Journal of Clinical Investigation,* **54,** 116–121
49. Piper, D.W., Glover, W.E. and Anthony, M. (1977). Cimetidine. *Current Therapeutics,* **18,** 11–16
50. Peatfield, R.C. and Rose, F.C. (1981). Ranitidine in migraine. *Annals of Neurology,* **10,** 61
51. Anthony, M., Lord, G.D.A. and Lance, J.W. (1978). Controlled trials of cimetidine in migraine and cluster headache. *Headache,* **18,** 261–264

52. Sicuteri, F. (1973). The ingestion of serotonin precursors (L-5-hydroxytryptophan and L-tryptophan) improves migraine headache. *Headache,* **13,** 19–22
53. Kangasniemi, P., Langvik, V-A. and Hyyppa, M.T. (1978). Levotryptophan treatment in migraine. *Headache,* **18,** 161– 166
54. Bono, G., Criscuoli, M., Martignoni, E., Salmon, S. and Nappi, G. (1982). Serotonin precursors in migraine prophylaxis. *Advances in Neurology,* **33,** 357–363
55. Stensrud, P. and Sjaastad, O. (1980). Comparative trial of Tenormin (atenolol) and Inderal (propranolol) in migraine. *Headache,* **20,** 206–207)
56. Biggs, R.S. and Millac, P.A. (1979). Timolol in migraine prophylaxis. *Headache,* **19,** 379–381
57. Stensrud, P. and Sjaastad, O. (1976). Short-term clinical trial of propranolol in racemic form (Inderal), d- propranolol and placebo in migraine. *Acta Neurologica Scandinavica,* **53,** 229–232
58. Diamond, S. and Medina, J.L. (1976). Double-blind study of propranolol for migraine prophylaxis. *Headache,* **16,** 24–27
59. Wideroe, T.E. and Vigander, T. (1974). Propranolol in the treatment of migraine. *British Medical Journal,* **2,** 699– 701
60. Ekbom, K. and Lundberg, P.O. (1975). Clinical trial of LB 46, an adrenergic-beta receptor blocking agent in migraine prophylaxis. *Headache,* **12,** 15–17
61. Ekbom, K. and Zetterman, M. (1977). Oxprenolol in the treatment of migraine. *Acta Neurologica Scandinavica,* **56,** 181–184
62. Ekbom, K. (1975). Alprenolol for migraine prophylaxis. *Headache,* **15,** 129–132
63. Yamamoto, M. and Meyer, J.S. (1980). Hemicranial disorder of vasomotor adrenoceptors in migraine and cluster headache. *Headache,* **20,** 321–335
64. Hansen, K.W., Klysner, R., Getsler, A., Knudsen, J.B., Glazer, S. and Gormsen, J. (1982). Platelet aggregation and beta-blockers. *Lancet,* **1,** 224–225
65. Weksler, B.B., Gillick, M. and Pink, J. (1977). Effect of propranolol on platelet function. *Blood,* **49,** 185–196
66. Fozard, J.R. (1982). Basic mechanisms of antimigraine drugs. In Critchley, M., Friedman, A.P., Gorini, S. and Sicuteri, F. (eds.) *Headache – Physiopathological and Clinical Concepts. Advances in Neurology,* **33,** 295– 307
67. Green, A.R. and Grahame-Smith, D.G. (1976). (– -Propranolol inhibits the behavioral responses of rats to increased 5-hydroxytryptamine in the central nervous system. *Nature,* **262,** 594–596
68. Middlemiss, D.N., Blakeborough, L. and Leather, S.R. (1977). Direct evidence for an interaction of β-adrenergic blockers with the 5-HT receptor. *Nature,* **267,** 289–290
69. Weinstock, N., Weiss, C. and Gitter, S. (1977). Blockade of 5-hydroxytryptamine receptors in the central nervous system by β-adrenoceptor antagonists. *Neuropharmacology,* **16,** 273–276
70. Lance, J.W. (1982). What is migraine? *Advances in Neurology,* **33,** 21–26
71. Anthony, M. (1981). Biochemical indices of sympathetic activity in migraine. *Cephalalgia,* **1,** 83–89
72. Anthony, M. (1982). Serotonin and cyclic nucleotides is migraine. *Advances in Neurology,* **33,** 45–49
73. Gomersall, J.D. and Stuart, A. (1973). Amitriptyline in migraine prophylaxis. Changes in pattern of attacks during a controlled clinical trial. *Journal of Neurology, Neurosurgery and Psychiatry,* **36,** 684–690
74. Couch, J.R., Ziegler, D.K. and Hassanein, R. (1976). Amitriptyline in the prophylexis of migraine. *Neurology,* **26,** 121–127
75. Lance, J.W. and Curran, D.A. (1964). Treatment of chronic tension headache. *Lancet,* **1,** 1236–1239
76. Baldessarini, R.J. (1980). Drugs and the treatment of psychiatric disorders. In Goodman and Gilman (eds.) *The Pharmacological Basis of Medical Practice.* 6th edition. New York: Macmillan, 391–447
77. Garattini, S. (1978). Platelet–drug interactions: an open field, in De Gaetano, G. and Garattini, S. (eds.). *Platelets: a Multidisciplinary Approach.* New York: Raven Press
78. Da Prada, M., Richards, J.G. and Ketti, R. (1981). Amine storage organelles in platelets. In Gordon, J.L. (ed.) *Platelets in Biology and Pathology, 2.* Amsterdam: Elsevier, 107–145

79. Kimball, R.W., Friedman, A.P. and Vallejo, E. (1960). Effect of serotonin in migraine patients. *Neurology,* **10,** 107–111
80. Anthony, M. and Lance, J.W. (1969). Monoamine oxidase inhibition in the treatment of migraine. *Archives of Neurology,* **21,** 263–268
81. Louis, P. (1981). A double-blind placebo-controlled prophylactic study of flunarazine (Sibelium^{R}) in migraine. *Headache,* **21,** 236–239
82. Louis, P. and Spierings, E.L.H. (1982). Comparison of flunarizine (Sibelium^{R}) and pizotifen (Sanomigran^{R}) in migraine treatment: A double-blind study. *Cephalalgia,* **2,** 197–203
83. Amery, W.K. (1983). Flunarizine, a calcium channel blocker: a new prophylactic drug in migraine. *Headache,* **23,** 70–74
84. Gelmers, H.J. (1983). Nimodipine, a new calcium antagonist, in the prophylaxis of migraine. *Headache,* **23,** 106–109
85. Meyer, J.S. and Hardenberg, J. (1983). Clinical effectiveness of calcium entry blockers in prophylactic treatment of migraine and cluster headache. *Headache,* **23,** 139
86. Solomon, G.D., Steel, J.G. and Spaccavento, L.J. (1983). Migraine prophylaxis with verapamil – a preliminary report. *Headache,* **23,** 139
87. Peroutka, S.J., Banghart, S.B. and Allen, G.S. (1983). Selectivity of calcium channel antagonists for intracerebral versus peripheral vascular smooth muscle. *Headache,* **23,** 138
88. Holmes, B., Brogden, R.N., Heel, R.C., Speight, T.M. and Avery, G.S. (1984). Flunarazine. A review of its pharmacodynamic and pharmacokinetic properties and therapeutic use. *Drugs*
89. Swanson, J.W. and Vick, N.A. (1978). Basilar artery migraine: 12 patients, with an attack recorded electroencephalographically. *Neurology,* **28,** 782–786
90. Eadie, M.J. and Tyrer, J.H. (1980). *Anticonvulsant Therapy. Pharmacological Basis and Practice.* 2nd edition. Edinburgh: Churchill-Livingstone
91. Glaser, G.H., Penry, J.K. and Woodbury, D.M. (eds.) (1980). *Antiepileptic Drugs. Mechanisms of Action.* New York: Raven Press
92. Couch, J.R. and Ziegler, D.J. (1978). Prednisone therapy for cluster headache. *Headache,* **18,** 219–221
93. Jammes, J.L. (1975). The treatment of cluster headache with prednisone. *Diseases of the Nervous System,* **316,** 375–376
94. Ekbom, K. (1981). Lithium for cluster headache: review of the literature and preliminary results of long-term treatment. *Headache,* **21,** 132–139
95. Peatfield, R.C. and Rose, F.C. (1981). Exacerbation of migraine by treatment with lithium. *Headache,* **21,** 140– 142
96. Okayasu, H., Meyer, J.S., Mathew, N.T., Amano, T. and Hardenberg, J. (1983). Lithium carbonate has no measurable effects on cerebral hemodynamics in cluster headache. *Headache,* **23,** 144
97. Curzon, G., Barrie, M. and Wilkinson, M.I.P. (1969). Relationships between headache and amine changes after administration of reserpine to migrainous patients. *Journal of Neurology, Neurosurgery and Psychiatry,* **32,** 555–561
98. Genefke, I.K., Dalsgaard-Nielsen, T., Bryndum, B., Fog-Moller, F. and Jensen, J.A.P. (1975). Concentration of serotonin in blood platelets: effect of reserpine in migraineurs. *Headache,* **15,** 136–141
99. Nattero, G., Lisino, F., Brandi, G., Gastaldi, L., Genefke, I.K. (1976). Reserpine for migraine prophylaxis. *Headache,* **15,** 279–281
100. Kaneko, Z., Shiraishi, J., Inaoka, H., Furukawa, T. and Sekiyama, M. (1978). Intra- and extracerebral hemodynamics of migrainous headache. In Greene, R. (ed.). *Current Concepts in Migraine Research.* New York: Raven Press, 17–24
101. Dalsgaard-Nielsen, T., Bryndum B., Fog-Moller F. and Genefke, I.K. (1974). The effect of percutaneous nitroglycerine upon the concentration of serotonin, epinephrine and norepinephrine in venous blood from migrainous subjects during attack-free intervals. *Headache,* **14,** 231–234
102. Kistler, J.P., Vielma, J.D., Davis, K.R., Fitzgibbon, S., Lees, R.S. and Crowell, P.M. (1982). Effects of nitroglycerine on the diameter of intracranial and extracranial arteries in monkeys. *Archives of Neurology,* **39,** 631–634
103. Schmidt, R. and Fanchamps, A. (1974). Effect of caffeine on intestinal absorption of ergotamine in man. *European Journal of Clinical Pharmacology,* **7,** 213–216

104. Saper, J.R. (1978). Migraine II. Treatment. *Journal of the American Medical Association,* **239,** 2480–2484
105. Hannington, E. (1980). Diet and migraine. *Journal of Human Nutrition,* **34,** 175–180
106. Rowsell, A., Neylan, C. and Wilkinson, M. (1973). Ergotamine-induced headache in migrainous patients. *Headache,* **13,** 65–67
107. Legg, N.J. (1976). Rebound migraine. *British Medical Journal,* **2,** 331
108. Anderson, P.G. (1974). Ergotamine headache. *Headache,* **15,** 118–121
109. Horton, B.T. (1941). The use of histamine in the treatment of specific types of headache. *Journal of the American Medical Association,* **116,** 377–383
110. Hanington, E., Horn, M. and Wilkinson, M. (1970). Further observations on the effects of tyramine. In Cochrane, A.L. (ed.). *Background to Migraine.* London: Heinemann, 113– 119
111. Seltzer, S. (1982). Foods, and food and drug combinations, responsible for head and neck pain. *Cephalalgia,* **2,** 111– 124
112. Egger, J., Carter, C.M., Wilson, J., Turner, M.W. and Soothill, J.F. (1983). Is migraine food allergy? A double- blind controlled trial of oligoantigenic diet treatment. *Lancet,* **2,** 865–869
113. Merrett, J., Peatfield, R.C., Rose, F.C. and Merrett, T.G. (1983). Food related antibodies in headache patients. *Journal of Neurology, Neurosurgery and Psychiatry,* **46,** 738–742
114. Brainard, J.B. (1981). Angiotensin and aldosterone elevation in salt-induced migraine. *Headache,* **21,** 222– 226

Part C
Migraine Pathogenesis

8

Hypotheses of the biochemical pathogenesis of migraine

*In the foregoing sections of this book we have attempted to set down the major clinical facts concerning migraine and have tried to interpret these data in terms of the altered tissue and organ function responsible for them. The more important hypotheses which attempt to explain migraine in terms of altered physiology have then been presented and assessed. Then individual biochemical changes so far described in migraine have been evaluated to see how adequately they can correlate with the hypotheses interpreting the disorder at the level of altered physiology. However, to the present stage, the biochemical changes have been dealt with only in an individual and rather piecemeal fashion. It is now time to consider the known biochemical changes as a whole and to assess the hypotheses which attempt to interpret migraine pathogenesis at a molecular level. *

The dominant direction of interest in certain migraine hypotheses lies in understanding the cause of the disorder or the provocation of attacks; in other hypotheses the concern resides in the mechanism of production of the manifestations of the disorder. Up to the present point in this book the main purpose has been to explain the mechanism of the disorder rather than its causation. We shall continue to give precedence to this intention until we have gone as far as we are able in this regard. Then we shall shift our main direction of interest toward the question of causation, and finally shall try to link hypotheses directed at interpreting mechanisms with those directed at interpreting causation. In such an attempt we shall inevitably repeat certain material contained in earlier sections of this book. However repetition appears unavoidable if this chapter is to be read as a self-contained whole without the need to turn repeatedly to earlier parts of the text.

8.1 HYPOTHESES OF THE MECHANISM OF MIGRAINE ATTACKS

As discussed in Chapter 2, the main lines of hypothesis of the pathogenesis of migraine see the attacks as having either a dominantly (a) vascular, or (b) neural mechanism.

8.1.1 Platelet–vascular hypotheses of the migraine mechanism

In simplistic terms, the conventional vascular hypotheses, dating back to at least 1872[1], seem to regard the mechanism of migraine as comprising the sequence of intracranial and extracranial arterial constriction, followed by intracranial and extracranial arterial dilatation[2]. The intracranial arterial constriction accounts for the neurological manifestations of the disorder, the extracranial dilatation for the headache, or at least the earlier phases of the headache. The other vascular elements in migraine are clinically silent. When the data are looked at critically, there is reasonably convincing evidence of intracranial arterial constriction in migraine. There is not so much evidence of subsequent consistently-present intracranial vasodilatation, though intracranial vascular calibre returns to normal after the constrictive phase. There is clear enough evidence of scalp arterial and venous dilatation during the earlier part of the headache phase of migraine. However the postulated premonitory scalp arterial constrictive changes are far from established as a general phenomenon, though they were recorded in two cases by Lund[3], while Wolff *et al.*[4], noted an increased frequency of superficial temporal artery constriction in the 24 hours preceeding migraine headache. In migraine it is possible that scalp capillary perfusion is decreased from the outset of the attack. This decreased perfusion may persist into the phase when scalp arteries and veins dilate, creating a set of circulatory phenomena which can be explained by Heyck's[5] postulate of precapillary arteriolar constriction with opening of scalp arterio-venous shunts. Thus the cranial circulatory changes of migraine appear to comprise:

(1) intracranial arterial constriction;
(2) possible scalp precapillary arteriolar constriction, occurring more or less synchronously with the intracranial constriction; followed by
(3) passing off of the intracranial constriction, sometimes followed by cerebral vasodilatation; and not necessarily at the same time,
(4) dilatation of scalp arteries and the corresponding draining veins, perhaps

with opening of arterio-venous shunts between these vessels.

How adequately do such changes explain the clinical phenomena of migraine?

8.1.1.1 The intracranial arterial constriction

At first sight local cerebral cortical ischaemia from intracranial arterial constriction would appear an adequate explanation for the neurological manifestations which may occur in migraine. However, there is not a great deal of published angiographic evidence demonstrating the occurrence of such arterial constriction, though when the changes have been shown they have sometimes been appropriately sited to explain the neurological manifestations. The earlier cerebral blood flow studies in classical migraine showed reasonably appropriately situated cerebral oligaemia to explain the neurological disturbances in the disorder. More recent studies from the Copenhagen school, using more refined flow measurement apparatus, have failed to demonstrate an adequate anatomical correspondence between site and degree of oligaemia and the pattern of neurological disturbance. Further, the pattern of spread of the oligaemia has been difficult to explain in terms of spasm of a single cerebral artery. The possibility has therefore been raised that the neurological manifestations of migraine may be of primary cerebral origin and that their progression, if not their inception, may be related to that ill-understood phenomenon, the spreading cortical depression of Leão. The spreading cortical oligaemia of migraine would then appear to be related to an extending disturbance of cortical function. Thus it would be a consequence, rather than a cause, of the neurological dysfunction of migraine. In Section 2.1.2 some evidence was adduced suggesting that the interpretation given immediately above may not necessarily be valid, at least in relation to the vascular changes Leão[6] observed. The older idea that focal brain ischaemia causes the neurological manifestation of migraine is consistent with the occasional occurrence of brainstem and optic and other cranial nerve disturbance during migraine attacks (abnormalities so sited anatomically as to be difficult to explain in terms of spreading cortical depression). This idea is also consistent with the occurrence of cerebral cortical infarction in migraine, a phenomenon established by the evidence of computerized tomographic radiological head scanning and, in at least two instances, by autopsy (see p. 23). Further, it is consistent with the fact that intake of vasodilating substances terminates the auras of migraine (Section 2.1.3). One would not expect vasodilators to influence Leão's spreading depression, unless this phenomenon is of ischaemic origin and due to vascular spasm.

Therefore, despite the recent data from ^{133}Xe regional cerebral blood flow studies, it appears to us that the preponderance of evidence still favours cerebral vascular spasm (perhaps shifting in site over the cortical arteries rather than remaining static at one site, and possibly involving vessels too small to be seen at angiography) as being the best explanation we have for the varied neurological manifestations of migraine.

8.1.1.2 Scalp precapillary arteriolar constriction

The evidence for the existence of this constriction is mainly indirect. However during the aura phase Lund[3] demonstrated superficial temporal artery narrowing on the side of the subsequent headache. It seems possible that any resulting scalp ischaemia may not necessarily be painful at first, though it may produce pain if it persists for long enough (see below).

8.1.1.3 Intracranial vasodilatation

Restoration of cerebral blood flow following oligaemia, whether or not there is local hyperaemia, might be expected to be associated with passing off of the neurological manifestations of the disorder, if the latter were due to ischaemia.

8.1.1.4 Scalp arterial and venous dilatation with persisting precapillary arteriolar constriction

There is some reason for believing that scalp vasodilatation in the presence of increased scalp capillary perfusion, as occurs in exercise and fever, is not painful. However, this is not the exact vascular situation that is thought to apply in migraine, where capillary perfusion appears decreased despite dilatation of the larger vessels. Possibly arterio-venous shunting of blood occurs in migraine. This would explain the scalp pallor, despite distended local arteries and veins. Experience with other disorders in human medicine gives no indication as to whether or not scalp arterial and venous dilatation in the presence of precapillary arteriolar constriction would be painful. If it is, it would be easy to see how an increased amplitude of tissue pulsation from vasodilatation might confer a throbbing element on the pain so produced (such throbbing often occurs in migraine headache). It seems possible that scalp tissue ischaemia resulting from decreased capillary blood flow may lead to the local production of pain-producing chemicals. This may be the factor that produces the headache of migraine. If so, scalp vasodilatation would appear a mere secondary event from the viewpoint of headache production, and would simply determine the character of the pain at one stage in the overall evolution of the headache mechanism.

8.1.2 Biochemical basis of the vascular hypotheses

The version of the vascular hypothesis of migraine set out immediately above is certainly not supported by conclusive evidence. Some of its elements are matters of inference rather than of proof, and vasodilatation is seen in a perhaps more subsidiary role than has been usual in the past. Nevertheless, for want of a better, it may serve as a reasonable operating hypothesis for which a biochemical basis should be sought.

8.1.2.1 The initial cerebral and extracranial arterial and/or arteriolar constriction

Serotonin Serotonin appears the best candidate yet indentified for a role in producing cerebral and scalp arterial constriction in the early phases of migraine. Its role in constricting cerebral arterioles is less certain[7] and we do not know its effect on scalp arterioles. There is experimental evidence (Section 3.1.1.4) that serotonin decreases cerebral, and probably extracranial, blood flow. The source of the serotonin that plays a role in migraine appears to be the circulating platelets. As was discussed in Section 2.2, prior to and during migraine circulating platelets show an increased tendency to form microaggregates. Platelet aggregation is a precursor to serotonin release. During migraine attacks platelets also appear to have a decreased capacity to take up serotonin. There appears to be compelling evidence of a decrease in platelet serotonin content during migraine attacks. The decrease in platelet serotonin level is usually of the order of 15–25%. If all this serotonin were released into plasma, and remained undegraded within the circulation, the released serotonin might increase plasma water serotonin concentration by a factor of perhaps 5 or 10. Since normal plasma water serotonin content is uncertain, the increase cannot be calculated more exactly. Even in the presence of ongoing serotonin biotransformation, the probable increase in plasma water serotonin concentration would appear sufficient to be likely to cause vasoconstriction. The reported increase in urinary excretion of 5-hydroxyindoleacetic acid during migraine, though not found in all studies, is consistent with metabolism of the released serotonin through the agency of the enzyme monoamine oxidase.

The above facts concerning platelets and serotonin form the basis of Hanington's suggestion[8,9] that migraine represents a primary platelet disorder. However in the present context we are concerned with hypotheses of migraine mechanisms. Hypotheses bearing on the cause and provocation of migraine will be considered later.

Catecholamines There are conflicting reports as to whether plasma noradrenaline levels rise[10] or fall[11] prior to migraine attacks. A rise in level at this time could contribute to, or cause, the vasoconstrictive phenomena of the earlier stages of migraine, whereas a fall in noradrenaline level would seem causally unrelated to these phenomena. Elevated noradrenaline concentrations during attacks (found by Fog-Muller *et al.*[11] and Anthony[12]) could maintain vasoconstriction. However these latter data cannot be interpreted in greater detail because information is lacking as to the time relationship between the catecholamine changes and the stage of evolution of the migraine attacks.

Eicosanoids Although thromboxane A_2 released from aggregating platelets would appear to be a potential contributing factor in the vasoconstrictive phase of migraine, so far no evidence appears to have been published demonstrating such thromboxane release.

As well as acting directly on vascular smooth muscle, circulating serotonin and noradrenaline (and any released thromboxane A_2) might promote platelet aggregation, leading to further local serotonin release, which in turn would favour further platelet aggregation.

Reported alterations in the concentrations of two circulating vasoactive amines (serotonin and noradrenaline) can go at least some distance toward explaining the vasoconstrictive phenomena of the earlier stages of migraine. Such alterations in circulating chemicals cannot of themselves explain why these vasoconstrictive changes may be localised to particular portions of the cerebral and scalp circulations. To explain this localised distribution of vascular alterations one must invoke some additional local circulatory abnormality which may vary in site from attack to attack, or even during the one attack. Alternatively, the local release of a potent vasoconstrictive agent with a transient existence could provide an explanation. Platelet thromboxane A_2 has properties which would qualify it for this latter role, though why platelets should release thromboxane A_2 only at certain points in the cranial circulation seems totally obscure unless platelet mobility was restricted. If there were some local abnormality which enabled serotonin and noradrenaline to have a greater effect in one part of the circulation than elsewhere, the resultant vasoconstriction might slow the local circulation, favour further platelet aggregation, and allow a high local thromboxane A_2 concentration to develop. This would initiate a self-perpetuating mechanism.

8.1.2.2 Scalp, and perhaps brain, vasodilatation

Is the arterial and venous dilatation that often occurs in parts of the scalp during the earlier stages of the headache phase of migraine merely a result of the passing off of prior vasoconstriction, or is the dilatation an active process? At first sight, one might assume that the lowered platelet serotonin concentrations that occur during migraine would after a time be associated with subnormal plasma water serotonin concentrations. This decrease in concentration of a circulating vasoconstrictor agent might produce vasodilatation. In the first place, there is as yet no proof that plasma water serotonin levels are reduced at any stage of migraine. Secondly, if the scalp circulation dilated during migraine in response to a decreasing serotonin effect there should be increased scalp capillary blood flow, and this does not seem to occur. Therefore depletion of circulating plasma water serotonin seems unlikely to explain the scalp vasodilatation of migraine. It is conceivable that plasma water serotonin concentrations could remain raised throughout much of an migraine attack, due to continuing leakage of serotonin from platelets. Because so much of the total plasma serotonin content is present in platelets, measurement of platelet or of whole plasma serotonin content might easily give little clue to a 2 or 3-fold increase in plasma water serotonin level during migraine, yet such an increase might have a very significant vasoconstrictive effect. One could then suggest that continuing scalp ischaemia from serotonin maintained vascular constriction (in a self-perpetuating mechanism as suggested above, with perhaps a contribution from noradrenaline and thromboxane A_2) might cause the local intravascular and perivascular release of vasodilator chemicals. These chemicals might then cause opening of scalp arterio-venous shunts, and arterial and venous dilatation, which would be maximal near the sites of vasodilator synthesis, since the vasodilator chemical concentrations would tend to be highest there. This secondary dilatation might occur in the presence of continuing serotonin or thromboxane A_2-maintained constriction of precapillary arterioles, particularly if the thromboxane had attained a high local concentration before vasodilator formation began. There would then be continuing scalp tissue ischaemia, ensuring a continuing production of the vasodilator molecules. Candidates for such a vasodilator role would include bradykinin, or a related kinin, and prostacyclin. Burnstock[13] suggested that adenosine triphosphate, the corresponding di-phosphates and mono-phosphates, and the purine base itself, might also be involved. These substances have appropriate properties for the role nominated. With the exception of the probable presence of kinins in the region of the scalp in which headache is experienced during attacks (Section 3.5.2), there is as yet no evidence that any of these substances is present in increased concentrations at the appropriate sites in migraine. It would be desirable to use modern chemical methods to confirm the presence of the kinins around scalp vessels during migraine. Local scalp vessel prostacyclin production has not been demonstrated during migraine, though such eicosanoid formation is known to occur in ischaemic endothelium. It would probably be difficult to detect scalp vascular prostacyclin formation from sampling of systemic venous blood. The eicosanoid has a transient existence and would be formed in a small volume of the circulation so that it might undergo considerable dilution by the time it reached peripheral veins.

If plasma water serotonin levels were to remain raised during the earlier part of the headache phase of migraine it is possible that serotonin might diffuse out through ischaemic, abnormally permeable, scalp capillary endothelium into perivascular spaces. Increased tissue serotonin concentrations, in the presence of bradykinin and perhaps certain prostaglandins, are known to be capable of producing pain. Adenosine, and its various phosphate derivatives, nominated for a role in migraine by Burnstock[13], also have nocioceptive actions. Thus the postulated formation of vasodilating chemicals as a result of scalp ischaemia could also explain headache production in migraine. Seen in this light the scalp vasodilatation of migraine would not be the cause of the head pain of the disorder, but would be a consequence of the chemical changes which themselves caused the pain and would confer on the pain its pulsatile character. In milder instances lesser quantities of dilator – algesic chemicals might form and the pain might never take on a pulsatile character. Clinically, one has the impression that it is the more severe migraine attacks which have the more definite pulsatile element to the head pain.

If scalp vasodilatation in migraine is a result of local tissue ischaemia, and is determined by local chemical changes, any intracranial vasodilatation that occurs in the disorder may similarly be a local chemically-mediated response to local cerebral ischaemia. If so, intracranial vasodilatation need not occur synchronously with the scalp vasodilatation since both changes would not be due to any common circulating chemical, but would arise from locally produced chemicals which could differ in nature and have different time courses of appearance. Burnstock[13] raised the possibility that adenosine and its various phosphates may play a vasodilator role intracranially in these circumstances.

It must be stressed that the above explanation contains in places a substantial element of speculation. Even if it is proved valid, the question still remains as to why the changes occur in a restricted anatomical distribution in the scalp and brain. In this regard, at least one clue is available. Migraine attacks sometimes begin in young or early middle-aged persons following minor blunt head injuries, injuries too minor to be likely to cause any significant brain damage. When this happens the migraine headaches commonly occur in that part of the scalp which has been injured. The attacks usually continue to occur, or at least to commence, in the same region of the scalp for months or years before they begin to appear in other areas. Could it be that injury to scalp tissues and local blood vessels in some way facilitates the biochemical reactions which lead to vasoconstriction and to kinin and eicosanoid formation? If so, in migraine widespread scalp and perhaps whole body arterial constriction produced by serotonin release from platelets into circulating plasma water might produce extensive but subclinical ischaemia, particularly in the affected scalp region. This ischaemia, in a scalp region predisposed to facile kinin and eicosanoid production, might then initiate a sufficiently intense local biochemical reaction to cause the pain and scalp vasodilatation of migraine.

In this way one would see the mechanism of the essential events of migraine as:

(1) Release of platelet serotonin, and perhaps discharge of noradrenaline into the circulation from sympathetic nervous system overactivity, cause vasoconstriction in the brain, scalp and elsewhere, with the serotonin and noradrenaline promoting further platelet activation with serotonin and thromboxane A_2 release.
(2) Because of local factors which are not understood, the brain vasoconstriction sometimes progresses in one cerebral region till manifestations of brain dysfunction appear: vasoconstriction may be more severe in one scalp region than in others, because of a local peculiarity of biochemical reaction. This vasoconstrictive phase persists until plasma water serotonin levels fall and/or some vasodilating substance formed locally (? prostacyclin, adenosine) overcomes the vasoconstriction.
(3) Because of local factors which might include a tendency to excessive formation of kinins and eicosanoids, plus leakage of serotonin through the ischaemic endothelium of sluggishly perfused scalp capillaries, the scalp ischaemia causes local pain in a portion of the scalp. Secondary dilatation of arteries and veins may then occur to a sufficient extent to impart a pulsatile character to the pain.
(4) The scalp pain neurally triggers posterior neck muscle contraction so that, as the local chemical disturbances in the scalp subside, muscle contraction headache comes to dominate the picture.
(5) If our own unpublished findings about platelet-rich plasma dopamine levels prove valid, increased plasma dopamine levels, produced in some as yet unknown way as a secondary phenomenon, may activate the medulla to cause nausea and vomiting: post-ischaemic reactionary conjunctival vasodilatation may make the eyes sensitive to light.

Thus the mechanism of the essential events of the migraine attack – the neurological disturbances, the headache, nausea, vomiting and photophobia –

might be explained. The above interpretation seems to us a fuller statement of the postulated biochemical events of the vascular – serotonin type hypothesis of migraine mechanisms than most of the versions which have been published, where the tendency has been to concentrate on one or other facet of the biochemical phenomena. As set down above, the hypothesis bears resemblance to Amery's[14] hypothesis that brain hypoxia (not necessarily due to ischaemia) is the turning point in determining whether or not clinical migraine occurs. The version of the hypothesis we have set down sees the intracranial and extracranial events of migraine as having a common initiation; thereafter they behave as largely independant variables biochemically and clinically, with degree of scalp ischaemia relative to degree of local biochemical peculiarity being the determinant of headache site and severity.

The above hypothesis may fit sufficient of the major clinical facts of migraine to appear beguiling. Nevertheless one must be very clear as to the extent to which it is based on intellectual leaps and inadequately proven, or completely non-existent, data. Thus, while there is reasonable evidence of platelet serotonin release, there is no direct proof that platelet-free plasma serotonin levels are raised during migraine attacks. Nor is the presence of brain and scalp vasoconstriction during migraine established beyond question. Local peculiarity in scalp vascular reactivity, at a physiological and a molecular level, is as yet a matter of inference, as is the postulated occurrence of scalp ischaemia and local production of nociceptive chemicals, with the exception of some rather ancient data concerning kinins. When the material is viewed critically, one would be justified in asking whether the available hard data warrant the proposal of any hypothesis at all. However, in science, some hypothesis nearly always proves better than none in allowing knowledge to advance. As we proceed to examine other biochemical hypotheses of migraine mechanisms the deficiencies in the vascular – serotonin hypothesis enunciated above may prove less than the deficiencies of its competitors.

8.1.3 Other circulation-centred hypotheses of migraine pathogenesis

8.1.3.1 Sandler's pulmonary hypothesis

Sandler[15] suggested that certain vasoactive substances, including serotonin and tryptamine, could cause the release of prostaglandins from the pulmonary vascular bed. He speculated that these prostaglandins might cause migraine by a systemic effect. Systemically administered prostaglandins in general undergo extensive degradation in the lungs. Therefore, for circulating prostaglandins to be able to act on the cerebral circulation to cause migraine, they would either have to by-pass the lungs or be formed in the lungs or in the circulation between the lungs and the head. The mechanism Sandler suggested thus provided a way for prostaglandins to reach the head and be involved in the pathogenesis of migraine.

Sandler's hypothesis lacked a foundation in experimental measurements of systemic arterial prostaglandin concentrations, and it was propounded before the existence of prostacyclin, a highly active prostaglandin not degraded by the lungs, was known. Sandler did not relate the postulated pulmonary release of prostaglandins to platelet serotonin release, and in fact concerned himself with the line of speculation that dietary tyramine might be the substance which activated pulmonary prostaglandin release. His hypothesis did not attempt to grapple with the detail of how the released prostaglandins would produce the various events of migraine.

Advances in knowledge, and lack of confirmatory experimental data in the years since it was proposed, have led to this hypothesis appearing progressively less attractive as time has passed.

8.1.4 Neurally-centred hypotheses

In essence, Sicuteri's[16] initial version of his central neurotransmitter serotonin depletion hypothesis attempted to explain pain production in migraine by providing a mechanism for pathological amplification of incoming pain impulses. The origin of the pain impulses was not made completely clear. Therefore it was possible to regard the earlier versions of the Sicuteri hypothesis as simply adding a pain- magnifying dimension to the traditional vascular hypothesis of the migraine mechanism. The relatively secondary role of the neurotransmitter serotonin depletion was brought out by the later suggestion that migrainous cerebral ischaemia was the cause of the fall in brain serotonin concentrations. In this light the central nervous serotonin events would be regarded as virtually an appendage to the traditional vascular hypothesis, though adding an additional dimension to it.

It would seem that Sicuteri came to recognise the possibility that the pain of migraine might arise centrally, and not merely be amplified centrally after arising elsewhere. This possibility opens the question of the neurological disturbances of migraine also being of endogenous neural rather than of ischaemic origin. If so, the vascular hypothesis becomes unnecessary and the vascular events that clearly do occur in migraine appear non-essential epiphenomena. As has been discussed earlier (Section 2.1.2), certain recently available evidence has called into question the adequacy of cerebral ischaemia as a basis for the neurological disturbances of migraine. On the other hand any postulated endogenous neural disturbance responsible for the neurological changes of migraine would be of quite unknown nature. A process akin to that of epilepsy does not seem an adequate explanation, for reasons given earlier (Section 2.3).

Lance[17] added to the basis of the Sicuteri central neurotransmitter depletion hypothesis by providing a more precise neuroanatomical background for the postulated neurotransmitter changes (Section 2.3). Lance looked to the neural control of the cerebral and extracranial circulations to suggest how altered function of a small zone in each side of the mid-brain and pons might produce unilateral intracranial and extracranial vascular changes in migraine, and might 'magnify' pain arising from these changes. Thus Lance explained unilateral headache (with a pulsatile character) and the vascular changes of migraine simultaneously. If the brain-stem disturbance he postulated was to become sufficiently restricted in its unilateral distribution it could be made to explain headache localised to part of one side of the head. Neurally-induced cerebral circulatory changes could explain the unilateral alterations in brain perfusion that have been demonstrated in some attacks of migraine. However, the question as to whether these changes cause the neurological disturbance, or whether this disturbance is of endogenous neural origin, is left unanswered.

Moskowitz and Coughlin[18] added to the detailed biochemical basis underlying this line of hypothesis by their suggestion that, in migraine, trigeminal nerve endings released vasoactive neurotransmitters around the large intracranial and extracranial blood vessels. The neurotransmitters they proposed for this role were the pain-producing vasodilating undecapeptide, substance P, and serotonin. They provided no evidence that such molecules were released in this way in migraine.

The above variants of the neurally centred hypothesis of the mechanism of migraine differ in the extent to which they see neurogenic events as predominating over vascular events in producing the manifestations of the disorder. None of the individual versions of this type of hypothesis really explains the production of the full gamut of the clinical features of the disorder, though Lance's version is perhaps the most satisfactory, and the most complete. However, once these hypotheses are looked at critically, one has to acknowledge that there is, as yet, no experimental evidence at all of a localised unilateral midbrain and pontine disturbance in migraine, no evidence of brain-stem serotonin depletion, and no evidence that trigeminal and facial nerve neurotransmitter release occurs in perivascular tissues, let alone causes vasodilatation. Thus the central tenets of these hypotheses are completely unproven. These neurally-centred hypotheses of the mechanism of migraine attacks stand largely by virtue of the known existence of a suitable anatomical and neurochemical background for their postulates, and by virtue of certain unsatisfactory features of the vascular-centered hypotheses, for which there is some experimental and observational evidence.

8.2 HYPOTHESES OF THE CAUSATION OF MIGRAINE

From the foregoing, one would probably conclude that, in the present state of knowledge, vascular-centred hypotheses of the mechanism of migraine appear more soundly based than neurally-centred hypotheses. No hypothesis of the cause (as distinct from the mechanism) of migraine is as yet based on anything like adequate experimental data. Hypotheses of the causation of migraine should interdigitate with hypotheses of the mechanism of migraine attacks. The more smoothly hypotheses at these two levels mesh, the more valid each hypothesis is likely to be. Therefore, as well as being important in its own right, a consideration of the mechanisms whereby migraine attacks may be instigated may add weight to one or other line of hypothesis of the mechanisms of migraine attacks.

Possible mechanisms through which various factors may initiate migraine attacks are dealt with in the following sections. It should be recognised that factors which activate the migraine mechanism may exert their influence hours or days before clinically recognizable migraine occurs, though there may be earlier clues that an attack is developing. Thus Tunis and Wolff[19] noted increased variability in the amplitude of the superficial temporal artery pulse up to 72 hours prior to the onset of migraine, suggesting that the vascular mechanism was becoming activated well before the sufferer was aware he had a migraine attack. If this is the case, it is possible that abortive subclinical migraine may occur.

8.2.1 Heredity

It seems widely accepted that some underlying tendency to migraine is familial, and probably inherited. The exact nature of what is inherited is unknown. It could be a tendency to altered cranial vascular reactivity, or to altered platelet behaviour, if vascular-type hypotheses are favoured. Alternatively, should neural-type hypotheses be preferred, it could be a peculiarity of regional midbrain and pontine function. In the absence of relevant experimental data there is little point in further consideration of this matter.

8.2.2 Emotional stress

Emotional stress, or sometimes the relief of such stress, is probably the most frequently identified provoker of migraine attacks. In a general intuitive way, one would expect that emotion would have its effect via altered central nervous system function. Emotion might activate the hypothalamus to produce sympathetic nervous system activity which could lead to peripheral noradrenaline (and dopamine-β-hydroxylase) release from nerve terminals, phenomena which are known to occur in migraine. Such a concept (as suggested by Johnson[20]) would link the method of attack initiation with a noradrenaline-mediated vascular type hypothesis of the migraine mechanism. Latham[1], suggested as much in 1872, though in ignorance of the molecular alterations now known to exist. It is only fair to point out that if emotion provoked migraine via noradrenaline release into the circulation, it becomes difficult to see how relief of emotional stress, which presumably diminishes peripheral sympathetic activity, could also provoke migraine by the same noradrenaline release mechanism. Clinically, migraine often follows relief of emotional stress. As an alternative possibility, it is conceivable that the anatomical substratum of emotion could project to the locus coeruleus via neural pathways. Thus there might be a connection between emotional factors which provoke migraine and neural-type hypotheses of the mechanism of migraine attacks. It is also possible that altered activity in the brain neural circuits that comprise the anatomical substratum of emotion may cause the release from the brain into the circulation of vasoactive, or platelet-active, chemicals. It seems likely that such chemical release would occur in regions where the blood–brain barrier was defective, such as in the hypothalamus. This type of proposal contains features of both neural and vascular hypotheses.

8.2.3 Sleep excess or insufficiency

Either lack of sleep, or sleeping too long, may produce migraine attacks in some individuals. The pattern of sleep would probably act at a central nervous system level to initiate migraine. It seems conceivable that altered reticular formation activity which may be associated with certain sleep patterns could, in some individuals, affect function in the locus coeruleus and nearby structures, though we do not know the precise anatomical pathways that would be involved.

Pineal indolealkylamine derivative levels show a diurnal rhythm in the circulation. The pineal lacks a blood – brain barrier. During sleep there is increased conversion of pineal serotonin into melatonin, *N*-acetyl serotonin and 5-methoxytryptamine (Section 3.1.1.3). Circulating levels of melatonin, at least, are substantially higher overnight than when awake. When an unusual pattern of sleep provokes migraine, it is possible that abnormal levels of these serotonin derivatives in the circulation affects vascular muscle function directly, or by altering platelet function. Melatonin is known to be capable of inducing migraine, even in the Parkinsonian age group, in whom migraine would ordinarily be uncommon[21]. Methoxytryptamine is known to be a potent constrictor of the human basilar artery[22]. It should be emphasised that such circulating indolealkylamine effects in migraine are as yet largely hypothetical, but the possibility of their occurrence warrants investigation. They could explain how a neural provocation of migraine acted via circulatory mechanisms.

8.2.4 Glare and dazzle

Exposure to glare and dazzle, or to intermittent intense light, may provoke migraine attacks in certain individuals. It is difficult to conceive that this activation of the disorder can be other than by neural mechanisms, when the process is instigated by light impinging on the retina and initiating impulses which traverse the visual pathway. It is known that light may simultaneously activate a pathway[23] which runs from the retina to the suprachiasmatic nucleus of the hypothalamus via the optic nerves. From the suprachiasmatic nucleus impulses pass along brain stem descending sympathetic pathways to the lower cervical and upper dorsal cord intermedio-lateral grey matter, then ascend the cervical sympathetic trunks to the superior cervical ganglia. Thence they pass through the pericarotid sympathetic plexuses, and via the nervi conarii synapse on pineal cells. Light impinging on the retina activates this highly circuitous pathway and results in ‘switching off’ of pinealocyte indolealkylamine metabolism, causing a fall in circulating melatonin levels. As explained above, there is no blood – brain barrier effect in the pineal. Therefore there is a known anatomical background for glare and dazzle to influence via neural mechanisms the function of a neuro – endocrine transducer which is involved in the production of vasoactive and platelet-active molecules. Perhaps the ‘switching-off’ of the mechanism by light exposure is somehow abnormal in certain migraine sufferers.

Of course, evidence is lacking that glare does activate migraine by involving this pathway to produce an abnormal pattern of secretion of pineal indoles into the circulation. The argument is simply that such a mechanism appears feasible. It might, in fairness, also be suggested that there could be an as yet undiscovered direct pathway from the suprachiasmatic nucleus to the midbrain raphe serotoninergic neuronal system, and that the whole mechanism of this variety of migraine production could be purely neural. Crook[24] did state that bright light caused central nervous system serotonin depletion.

8.2.5 Diet

Various items of food, and certain forms of alcohol, may induce attacks in some individuals with migraine[25]. So many different foods are involved, each composed of a variety of chemical molecules, that it becomes impracticable to assess the role of these individual substances in causing migraine attacks.

The role of certain dietary amines, tyramine and phenylethylamine, in provoking migraine has been the subject of some investigation. The action of these amines, if they escape degradation by monoamine oxidase in the alimentary tract epithelium, has generally been interpreted in terms of their capacity to displace serotonin from its stores in platelets, thus initiating a serotonin-vascular type of migraine mechanism. The possibility also arises as to whether these amines could act on central nervous system serotoninergic pathways to displace the neurotransmitter competitively and thus to produce central serotonin depletion. On first principles this possibility seems unlikely, since one would anticipate the circulating amines would be too polar to cross the blood – brain barrier, though phenylethylamine is said to be capable of crossing the barrier[26]. The amines might enter the pineal and, if they did, any displaced serotonin and other amines would presumably enter the circulation. It would appear that the provocation of migraine might correlate with either the vascular type of hypothesis of migraine mechanism or the neural type of hypotheses of the mechanism in the case of phenylethylamine. In the case of tyramine the better correlation would be with the vascular type hypothesis.

Going without food may also provoke migraine attacks in some persons. It seems clear that hypoglycaemia is not the causative mechanism in this situation. Because of the likely variation in chemical constitution of the diet from meal to meal it is awkward to argue that the absence of some specific dietary chemical can provoke attacks in certain persons when one also wishes to argue that attacks may be caused in other individuals by the intake of particular dietary chemicals. Possibly hunger simply acts as a stress, utilizing the same neural mechanisms as stress involves, whatever these mechanisms may be.

8.2.6 Falling oestrogen concentrations

The tendency to the premenstrual occurrence of migraine, the deferment of these attacks by oestrogen therapy, the propensity of oestrogen-containing oral contraceptives to cause migraine, and the frequent disappearance of the disorder during pregnancy (with its high oestrogen concentrations), all suggest that a fall in circulating oestrogen concentration can precipitate migraine in women. The mechanisms involved are unclear. Oestrogens may affect receptors in the hypothalamus, and by this route could alter nervous system function. Unfortunately the precise anatomical pathways by which the postulated hypothalamic alteration could affect the locus coeruleus and its surrounds are uncertain. Oestrogens do alter arachidonate metabolism, and thus might affect platelet function in migraine, but this connection is no more than a matter of inference.

Not enough is known of the mechanisms of oestrogen action to explain oestrogen-related migraine adequately. Consequently, little light is thrown on mechanisms likely to be involved in provoking migraine attacks.

8.2.7 Certain drugs

8.2.7.1 Reserpine

Reserpine can activate migraine attacks. The drug causes amine storage granules in both platelets and nerve terminals to fail to retain their amine contents. Thus reserpine can initiate the set of platelet-mediated serotonin-related events which are the central tenets of the serotonin–vascular hypothesis of the migraine mechanism. Equally, reserpine could account for central neurotransmitter serotonin depletion, following initial leakage of stored serotonin into synapses. Reserpine should also deplete catecholamine neurotransmitter stores, again with initial increased synaptic leakage. Whether drug-induced initial leakage of noradrenaline and serotonin, which temporarily raises amine concentrations at perivascular nerve endings, could explain cerebral vasoconstrictive events in migraine attacks, with subsequent neurotransmitter depletion causing both vasodilatation and pain potentiation, is uncertain. One would need more information about the durations of the various postulated phenomena.

8.2.7.2 Glyceryl trinitrate (nitroglycerine)

Glyceryl trinitrate (nitroglycerine) sometimes produces a short-lived pulsatile headache. It is known to activate attacks of migrainous neuralgia during clusters, and also migraine. The drug is a potent vasodilator without known action on the central nervous system when given in therapeutic dosage. Therefore its known mechanism of action suggests that it probably provokes migraine by a direct vascular effect.

8.2.8 Migraine provocation – an overview

It seems probable that certain of the factors which can activate migraine do so by virtue of a vascular (or platelet)-directed effect. Such factors include certain dietary amines (tyramine) and glyceryl trinitrate. On the other hand certain other migraine precipitants (such as stress or glare) almost certainly exert their initial effects on the nervous system. In migraine attacks it is possible that an initial vascular change could alter brain blood flow to produce a secondary alteration in nervous system function. This could then set in train the neural mechanisms responsible for the clinical manifestations of migraine. It is also possible that primarily neural mechanisms of migraine provocation could cause the release of vasoactive and platelet active substances from the hypothalamus or pineal into the circulation. This release would set the stage for the events of the vascular–serotonin type hypothesis of the mechanism of migraine attacks.

What seems clear from this consideration is that neither solely neural or solely vascular events can explain the full gamut of the phenomena of migraine and its provocation. There must be interaction between the dysfunctions of the two systems, though the level and direction of the interaction remain uncertain. It may be necessary to consider the possibility of interaction at two levels, for example a migraine precipitant first acting on the nervous system to cause release of vasoactive chemicals, with these chemicals then acting within the circulation to reduce regional cerebral blood flow, thus producing the neurological disturbance of 'classical' migraine.

Plainly, knowledge of the various possible biochemical changes involved in the precipitation of migraine attacks provides no decisive basis for preferring vascular – platelet – serotonin type hypotheses of the mechanism of migraine to neurally-centred hypotheses of this mechanism.]*

8.3 BIOCHEMICAL PATHOGENESIS OF MIGRAINE

Hypotheses of the biochemical background to migraine, and of the production of attacks, should be linked to hypotheses of the biochemical mechanisms of migraine attacks to yield an overall hypothesis of the pathogenesis of the disorder. Before this can be done it is necessary to settle on a general line of preferred hypothesis for the mechanism of migraine attacks. In our view, in the present state of knowledge the vascular – serotonin type of hypothesis is to be preferred to neurally-central hypotheses. Despite some admittedly unsatisfactory aspects, there is at least some direct observational evidence obtained during migraine attacks in favour of the vascular-centred hypothesis, while similar evidence for neural-type hypotheses is totally lacking. Further, known mechanisms of action of drugs which benefit migraine fit better with the vascular – serotonin hypotheses than the neural ones. Unsatisfactory as they may seem, such are the reasons for our preference.

* [The best hypothesis of migraine pathogenesis that we can advance divides the matter into three levels:

(1) the underlying predisposition
(2) the factors that precipitate attacks
(3) the final common pathway – the mechanism of the attacks.

(1) The predisposition to migraine appears genetic, or at least familial. The biochemical basis, and the molecular mechanisms at which it expresses itself, are completely unknown.

(2) The precipitating factors may (a) act directly on platelet and/or vessel wall mechanisms, or (b) act indirectly, via sympathetic nervous system-mediated changes in vascular tone and via noradrenaline release into the circulation, or perhaps via release of vasoactive and platelet-active substances from the hypothalamus and/or pineal.

(3) The final common pathway, in which platelet serotonin and perhaps thromboxane A_2 release causes vasoconstriction, particularly affects predisposed intracranial and extracranial vascular beds. The cerebral ischaemia so produced may cause focal neurological dysfunction. The

extracranial soft tissue ischaemia so produced may cause local release of vasodilator and pain-producing chemicals such as kinins, prostacyclin and other eicosanoids, which together with serotonin which leaks into the scalp, causes local head pain. This headache, via neural reflexes, triggers (potentially self-perpetuating) neck muscle contraction headache, the late-stage element in the pain production.

The above (shown in Figure 8.1) is the skeleton of the best hypothesis we can construct in terms of the knowledge we have available. Flesh can be added to some of the bones of the hypothesis by using material that we have already discussed, for example data concerning the precipitation of attacks, the question of post-ischaemic vasodilatation,the possible role of dopamine in producing nausea and vomiting. One could speculate that brain – stem ischaemia in the final common pathway stage could lead to central neurotransmitter serotonin depletion, and thus amplification of pain initiated by a quite different peripheral vascular mechanism. Proposing a hypothesis such as that set down above should simply serve as a stimulus for others to attack it, modify it or demolish it, their efforts being based on experimental data not currently available to us, or on more clear-sighted reason.

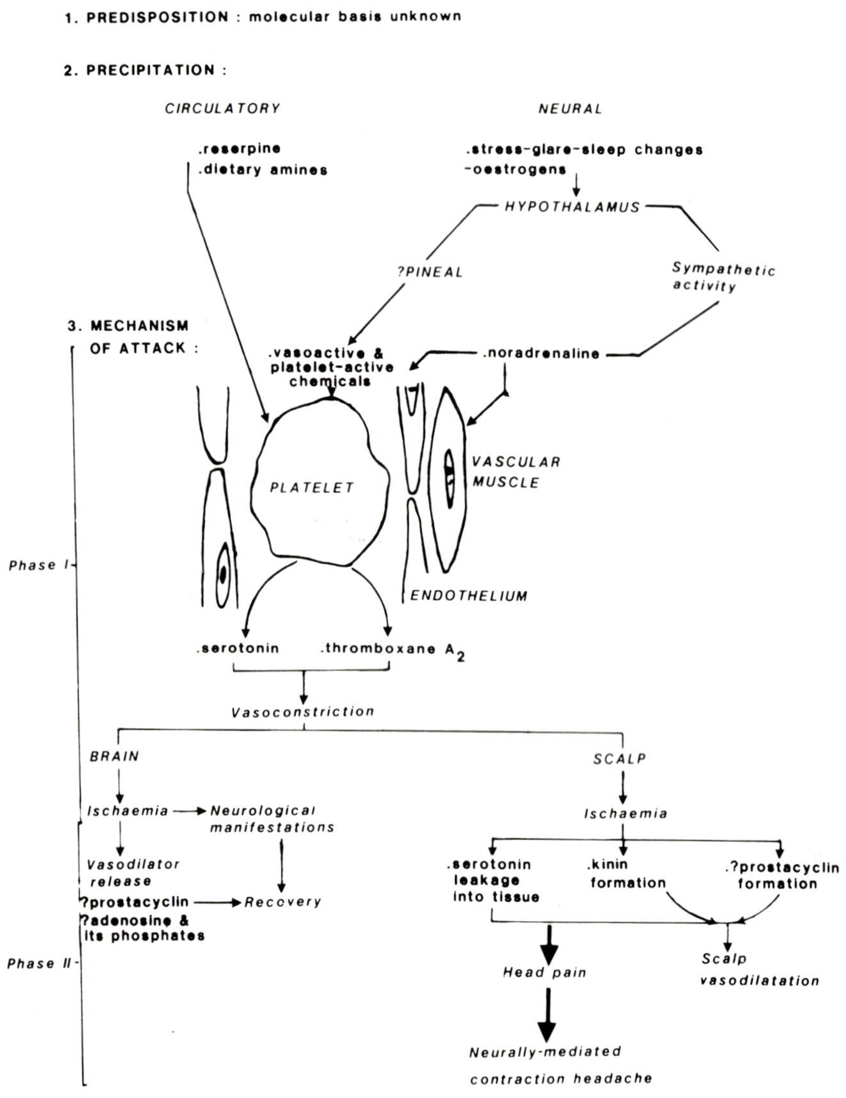

Figure 8.1 Hypothesis of the pathogenesis of migraine

References

1. Latham, P.A. (1892). Clinical lectures on nervous or sick headaches. *British Medical Journal,* **1,** 305–306; 336–337
2. Brazil, P. and Friedman, A.P. (1956). Craniovascular studies in headache: a report and analysis of pulse volume tracings. *Neurology,* **6,** 96–102
3. Lund, F. (1957). Studies on the shape of the temporal artery pulsations in vascular headache, particularly migraine. *Acta Medica Scandinavica,* **158,** 21–34
4. Wolff, H.G., Tunis, M.M. and Goodell, H. (1953). Studies on headache. Evidence of tissue damage and changes in pain sensitivity in subjects with vascular headaches of the migraine type. *Archives of Internal Medicine,* **92,** 478–484
5. Heyck, H. (1970). The importance of arteriovenous shunts in the pathogenesis of migraine. In Cochrane, A.L. (ed.) *Background to Migraine.* London: Heinemann, 19–35
6. Leão, A.A.P. (1944). Pial circulation and spreading depression of activity in the cerebral cortex. *Journal of Physiology,* **7,** 391–396
7. Van Nueten, J.M. (1983). 5-Hydroxytryptamine and precapillary vessels. *Federation Proceedings,* **42,** 223–227
8. Hanington, E. (1978). Migraine: a blood disorder? *Lancet,* **2,** 501–503
9. Hanington, E. (1982). Migraine as a blood disorder: preliminary studies. *Advances in Neurology,* **33,** 253–256
10. Hsu, L.K.G., Crisp, A.H., Kalucy, R.S., Koval, R.S., Chen, C.N., Carruthers, M. and Zilkha, K.J. (1977). Early morning migraine. Nocturnal plasma levels of catecholamines, tryptophan, glucose, and free fatty acids and sleep encephalographs. *Lancet,* **1,** 447–451
11. Fog-Moller, F., Genefke, I.K. and Bryndum, B. (1978). Changes in the concentration of catecholamines in blood during spontaneous migraine attacks and reserpine-induced attacks. In Greene, R. (ed.) *Current Concepts in Migraine Research.* New York: Raven Press, 115–119
12. Anthony, M. (1981). Biochemical indices of sympathetic activity in migraine. *Cephalalgia,* **1,** 83–89
13. Burnstock, G. (1981). Nervous control of cerebral blood vessels: a new hypothesis for the mechanisms underlying migraine. In Rose, F.C. and Zilkha, K.J. (eds.) *Progress in Migraine Research. 1.* London: Pitman, 17–32
14. Amery, W.K. (1982). Brain hypoxia: the turning-point in the genesis of the migraine attack. *Cephalalgia,* **2,** 83–109
15. Sandler, M. (1972). Migraine: a pulmonary disease? *Lancet,* **1,** 618–619
16. Sicuteri, F. (1972). Headache as a possible expression of deficiency of brain 5-hydroxytryptamine (central denervation supersensitivity). *Headache,* **12,** 69–72
17. Lance, J.W. (1981). Headache. *Annals of Neurology,* **10,** 1–10
18. Moskowitz, M.A. and Coughlin, S.R. (1981). Basic properties of the prostaglandins. *Stroke,* **12,** 696–701
19. Tunis, M.M. and Wolff, H.G. (1954). Studies on headache: cranial artery vasoconstriction and muscle contraction headache. *Archives of Neurology and Psychiatry,* **71,** 425–434
20. Johnson, E.S. (1978). A basis for migraine therapy – the autonomic theory reappraised. *Postgraduate Medical Journal,* **54,** 231–242
21. Papavasaliou, P.S., Cotzias, G.C., Duby, S.E., Steck, A.J., Bell, M. and Lawrence, W.H. (1972). Melatonin and Parkinsonism. *Journal of the American Medical Association,* **221,** 88–89
22. Forster, C. and Whalley, E.T. (1981). Comparison of the contraction produced by various tryptamine analogues on human basilar arterial and rat aortic strips in vitro. *Cephalalgia,* **1,** 217–221
23. Reiter, R.J. (1981). The mammalian pincal gland: structure and function. *American Journal of Anatomy,* **162,** 287–313
24. Crook, M. (1981). Migraine: a biochemical headache? *Biochemical Society Transactions,* **9,** 351–357
25. Hanington, E. (1980). Diet and migraine. *Journal of Human Nutrition,* **34,** 175–180
26. Oldendorf, W.H. (1971). Brain uptake of radiolabelled amino acids, amines and hexoses after arterial injection. *American Journal of Physiology,* **221,** 1629–1639

9
The future – what might usefully be done

From the contents of the foregoing chapters, it is obvious that our understanding of the pathogenesis of migraine is far from complete. Those who practise clinical neurology will be equally aware that our ability to treat the disorder often proves unsatisfactory, despite use of the available drugs in a manner that appears optimal in terms of contemporary pharmacokinetic and pharmacodynamic knowledge. The best strategy for more effective treatment of migraine seems to lie in obtaining a more complete understanding of the biochemistry of the disorder, and then using this knowledge to devise more efficient therapies.

The present chapter attempts to suggest some lines of investigation which appear potentially fruitful in filling certain gaps in our understanding of the pathogenesis of migraine. These gaps have become apparent when considering the matters dealt with in earlier sections of this book. The suggested lines of investigation are mainly concerned with deficiencies in the vascular – serotonin type of hypothesis of migraine mechanism. The reason for this apparent bias lies in the fact that there is no animal model of migraine available for laboratory investigation. The physiological and biochemical basis of migraine must therefore be studied in human sufferers. In man it would be virtually impossible, and certainly ethically unacceptable, to carry out direct investigations of the postulated brain-stem chemical changes underlying the neurally-centred hypothesis of the disorder. However, it is quite feasible, and ethically justifiable, to investigate many aspects of the vascular-type hypotheses; such investigations often merely involve sampling of peripheral blood. The most practicable approach may therefore be to investigate the mechanisms of various elements of the vascular – serotonin hypothesis, modifying the hypothesis as necessary and, when enough evidence accumulates, to decide whether the hypothesis stands or falls. If it falls, one will then have to face the difficult task of direct investigation of the neural type of hypothesis, or of any apparently viable alternative interpretation.

9.1 INVESTIGATIONS AT A CLINICAL LEVEL

One of the problems in investigating migraine at a clinical level is involuntary bias in respect to the patients selected for study. Almost inevitably those who are in a position to collect sufficient cases of migraine for any sort of statistical study (for example neurologists, researchers working in headache or pain clinics) tend to see a selected group of migraineurs. In particular they see those with more severe or more frequently-occurring forms of the disorder, or those with unusual manifestations. It is therefore possible that the picture of migraine described in conventional textbooks may have come to portray the more severe migraine sufferer, and may not faithfully represent an undistorted version of the average sufferer from the disorder. We can see that useful information might be obtained from studies carried out on large series of migraineurs, as will be suggested below. Such studies would probably be based on case records collected by those with a special interest in the disorder. We believe it could prove a valuable corrective, helping to keep the matter in valid perspective, if one or two such studies were also done in a collection of migraineurs drawn at random from a field survey of the prevalence of migraine in representative communities.

There are a number of clinical matters concerning migraine which we see as not adequately documented. In relation to these matters, it seems to us that well-founded data could open the way to fruitful biochemical investigation. These matters include the following:

(1) The course of migraine often extends over much of a given individual's life- span. Every neurologist will be aware that the manifestations in the individual often do not remain static over the years, and that, at certain stages in their lives, individuals may experience two or more recognizably different patterns of migrainous symptoms in different headache attacks. If clinical manifestations are not the same in different attacks, the underlying altered biochemistry may also differ between attacks. If we are to have a sound basis against which the biochemistry of migraine is to be interpreted we need better statistical data on the behaviour of the disorder with time in the affected individual's life. Careful statistical study may permit the definition of various subtypes of migraine attack (as has already been done without, on the whole, much statistical data being published to give quantitative perspective to the classification). Such study may also permit definition of subtypes of migraineurs, which might prove very illuminating when considering the question of the biochemical basis of the predisposition to migraine.

(2) We need additional detailed statistical data on the frequency of various clinical manifestations in migraine attacks, and in migraineurs,for example how often there is an aura, how long it lasts, in what percentage of a given individual's attacks does it occur, how often is the headache 'throbbing' in character, how frequently do nausea, vomiting and photophobia

occur. These data provide a necessary background for assessing how representative are the migraine attacks which occur in a small group of sufferers of attacks of migraine in general. Most biochemical investigations in migraine are done, of necessity, in groups of ten or twenty subjects, and if the attacks studied are not representative misleading inferences may be drawn.

(3) A cross-correlation (perhaps along the lines attempted by Diehr *et al.*[1]) between the presence of various patterns of symptom in migraine attacks and in migraineurs, and certain factors (such as age, sex, blood pressure, past history of illness or birth difficulty, nature of circumstances provoking attacks) may open new directions for biochemical research, or cause such research to be more appropriately focused.

(4) The factors precipitating migraine should be assessed critically, both as to their validity as precipitants, and as to the frequency with which such precipitation occurs. This information may prevent waste of effort in investigating unlikely clues with elaborate biochemical studies, and may permit the intensified channelling of effort towards promising and quantitatively important leads. Thus, for example, as may well be the case, if alcohol intake were shown to precipitate migraine attacks in, say, 25% of migraineurs, and intake of red wine were ten times as likely as intake of white wine to instigate the attacks, it would seem obvious that the difference in chemical constitution between red and white wine might be a rewarding preliminary field for investigation.

9.2 INVESTIGATION AT A PHYSIOLOGICAL LEVEL

Investigation on humans carried out at a tissue or an organ level is likely to take place in a hospital or similar environment. On the whole, it is likely to be carried out in persons whose migraine causes them to reach such an institution. These persons are therefore likely to represent a selected group of migraineurs. Findings obtained by studying them should be assessed in relation to the considerations discussed immediately above (Section 9.1).

More than anyone else Wolff, with his various co-workers, made the critical physiological observations which form the basis of much of our interpretation of the phenomena of migraine attacks[2]. Some of these observations need confirmation by more modern techniques, others need extension. Repeating some, it may be suspected, could trouble contemporary committees concerned with the ethics of research on humans. In all such studies, necessarily involving small groups of subjects, one should be clear as to how representative the sample is of the disorder as a whole. It would also be highly important to relate the physiological findings to the clinical manifestations extant at the time of the observations, if the investigations were carried out during migraine attacks. The possibility of abortive subclinical migraine during the apparent headache-free period in migrane sufferers should be borne in mind as a possible confounding factor in certain control studies.

Work which might usefully be done to clarify certain issues, and which appears practicable, includes the following:

(1) Sequential observations in a number of subjects throughout migraine attacks, commencing as early as possible in the attacks or even before their onsets, in relation to:
   (a) the pulsation of all accessible scalp arteries, and the carotid arteries in the neck;
   (b) the degree of posterior neck muscle and scalp muscle contraction, recorded electromyographically;
   (c) the scalp skin temperature at different sites;
   (d) the effect on the pain of local temporary occlusion of single and multiple arteries (the extent of the occlusion being confirmed by pulse recordings);
   (e) the effect on the pain of producing unilateral neck muscle relaxation by infiltrating the motor points of the relevant muscles with low concentrations of local anaesthetic capable of interfering with γ but not α motoneuron function (compared with control saline injections).

The above observations, made in a sufficient number of subjects at different stages of attacks, should help clarify the roles of scalp vasodilatation and neck muscle contraction in pain production.

(2) Repeating the observations listed under(1) immediately above in the same subject in several different migraine attacks to see how consistently present the mechanisms are.
(3) Carrying out regional cerebral flow studies, preferably using inhaled ^{133}Xe, or ^{133}Xe administered selectively via femoral catheter into the carotid system, and possibly the vertebro-basilar system during *spontaneous* migraine attacks. Such studies should be repeated at different stages of the attacks, and correlated with the clinical findings. An attempt should also be made to measure external carotid blood flow during different stages of migraine attacks.
(4) Carrying out sequential positron emission tomographic studies of regional cerebral glucose metabolism at stages of migraine attacks.
(5) Recording continuous scalp EEG's throughout the course of migraine attacks, and correlating the site and degree of any focal EEG changes which might develop with the clinical findings, and the situation revealed by various special investigations.
(6) Endeavouring to obtain fortuitous angiographic studies during spontaneous migraine attacks. Information obtained from angiographic studies done when the migraine develops following carotid puncture may be less valuable.
(7) Sequential computerized tomographic or proton magnetic resonance head scans during migraine attacks may or may not be illuminating, but the possibilities of these investigations should be explored.

If several of the above procedures could be carried out simultaneously in the one subject and the data correlated, the value of the investigation might be considerably enhanced. It is realized that simultaneous employment of the various items of apparatus involved in such studies may be impracticable for both technical and financial reasons. However, it should always be possible to correlate whatever observations can be made with carefully collected clinical data.

9.3 INVESTIGATIONS AT A BIOCHEMICAL LEVEL

One of the problems in interpreting much of the previous biochemical work on migraine is that it seems to have been carried out without regard to the stage of the attack at which the observations were made, almost as if it were believed that a single biochemical alteration might explain a number of changing clinical and physiological manifestations. When observations have been made on migraineurs between attacks it sometimes seems to have been tacitly assumed that all migraineurs are created biochemically equal and the possibility of subclinical attacks has been ignored. In future biochemical investigations on migraine we would suggest that care should be taken to:

(1) assess how representative the subject sample is of the disorder as a whole, or of one or other of its subtypes;
(2) correlate biochemical changes with the phase of evolution of the attacks;
(3) consider the possibility that studies carried out between attacks may sometimes be carried out during subclinical attacks, or in the chemical prodromes of attacks;
(4) consider the possibility that there may be clinical sub-types of migraine sufferer which correlate with certain biochemical phenomena in the intervals between attacks.

As with studies on migraine carried out at a physiological level, biochemical studies may be more illuminating and more reliable if performed sequentially during the course of migraine attacks, and repeated in several attacks in the same subject. Further, sequential blood and biological fluid sampling poses far less technical and financial problem than simultaneous access to the multiple bulkly, highly expressive, items of equipment that may be required for physiological studies. It should therefore often be feasible to measure a number of biochemical parameters simultaneously during attacks. Clearly, an admixture of such sequential biochemical studies with a judicious selection of physiological level investigations carried out at the same time in the same subject may offer an increased dimension of insight into the disorder. A deal of contemporary thinking about migraine is centred on platelet behaviour. We would therefore plead that, when relevant, future biochemical work on the disorder should differentiate very carefully between the concentrations of substances in platelets, and in platelet-free plasma (acknowledging the difficulty of preparing the latter without injuring platelets and thus contaminating the plasma with their contents).

The lines of biochemical investigation we see as potentially rewarding include the following:

(1) Sequential studies of platelet and platelet-free plasma levels of
    (a) serotonin,
    (b) noradrenaline,
    (c) adrenaline,
    (d) dopamine,

  (e) the pineal indoles, such as 5-methoxytryptamine, *N*-acetylserotonin, melatonin, taking into consideration the possible circadian rhythm of these substances, and of serotonin.

(2) Studies of plasma concentrations and urine excretions of metabolites of the above substances, including both primary metabolites and metabolite conjugates,such as:
  (a) 5-hydroxyindoleacetic acid and its glucuronide(s),
  (b) methoxyhydroxyphenylglycol and vanillylmandelic acid and their conjugates,
  (c) metanephrine,
  (d) homovanillic acid and dopamine sulphate,
  (e) the interplay between the numerous pineal indole metabolites may be too complex to yield easily interpretable answers.

(3) Sequential studies of platelet monoamine oxidase activity throughout migraine attacks and in different subtypes of migraine, and of migraineurs, to see if the reported monoamine oxidase changes can be substantiated.

(4) sequential studies of platelet and vascular wall eicosanoid production. The vessel wall eicosanoid production studies may require jugular venous blood sampling. Urinary eicosanoid metabolite excretion studies may provide supporting evidence.

(5) Sequential studies of circulating bradykinin levels during the course of migraine attacks.

(6) Sequential studies of circulating and, if feasible and ethically justifiable, cerebrospinal fluid opioid levels during the course of migraine attacks, using specific assays.

(7) Controlled sequential studies of at least the following substances in scalp tissue fluid during the course of unilateral migraine:
  (a) serotonin,
  (b) bradykinin and related kinins,
  (c) various eicosanoids,
  (d) adenosine itself and its phosphate esters,
  (e) substance P.

Experience may show that repeated scalp needling to obtain tissue fluid during a single migraine attack may itself promote the formation of some of these substances locally. Control sampling from the unaffected side will not exclude this possibility on the affected side, so that the interpretation of data may have to depend on single scalp samples taken at different stages in different attacks from a number of sufferers.

(8) A systematic attempt should be made to identify the unknown circulating factor which alters the behaviour of migraineurs' platelets. Once identified, the time course of the presence in plasma of this factor should be defined, both during and between migraine attacks.

The above proposed programme involves only substances known or suspected of being involved in migraine. Its implementation would involve a prodigious amount of laboratory work. Unquestionably, other investigations of the biochemistry of substances germane to an understanding of migraine could be done. While such investigations were underway it is highly likely that other substances (such as the oligopeptide neurotransmitters, the lipo-oxygenase derivatives of the eicosanoids and possibly the phenolic amines) will appear as stronger candidates for a role in the molecular pathology of migraine. At the worst, the very major programme of biochemical endeavour suggested above might achieve no more than a debunking of the vascular-serotonin type hypotheses of migraine pathogensis. Yet even this would be useful, in that it could divert research into potentially more rewarding channels.

Migraine is a major source of (generally intermittent) disability in the community. We do not understand it adequately, but for many years most workers appear to have been reasonably content with making piecemeal clinical, physiological and biochemical observations on it. On the basis of this very fragmentary and sometimes ambiguous knowledge we have been prepared to construct elaborate hypotheses of what might be happening in the disorder. Surely the time has come for a sustained systematic study to make or break what seems the most promising and best founded of these lines of hypothesis, with the ultimate aim of providing a basis for better treatment for sufferers from the disorder.

References

1. Diehr, P., Diehr, G., Koepsell, T., Wood, R., Beech, K., Wolcott, B. and Tomkins, R.K. (1982). Cluster analysis to determine headache types. *Journal of Chronic Diseases,* **33,** 623 – 633
2. Wolff, H.G. (1963). *Headache and Other Head Pains. 2nd edition.* New York: Oxford University Press

Part D
Cluster Headache

10
Cluster headache – migrainous neuralgia

It could be argued with some justification that it is inappropriate to consider the topic of cluster headache in a book on the biochemistry of migraine. However the clinical similarities between cluster headache and migraine are obvious. A generation ago there seems to have been a tendency to regard cluster headache merely as a migrainous variant, whereas contemporary nosological thinking tends to distance the two entities rather more. This increased distinction between the two disorders rests, in part, on biochemical data which have become available in the past two decades[1]. In fact some workers have tended to study cluster headache sufferers to obtain a 'group of patients to serve as a pain experiencing control group for comparison with migraineurs'. We have elected to deal with the subject of cluster headache in this book not because we see the disorder as an expression of a modified migraine mechanism but because, with its obvious clinical resemblances to certain aspects of migraine, it can be useful at times to argue from its mechanisms to the mechanisms of migraine. However, we have chosen to deal with cluster headache as an entity in a separate chapter whereas, if we regarded it as a modified migraine, it would have been more logical to deal with it in stages beside various appropriate aspects of migraine.

10.1 CLINICAL PHENOMENA

The clinical features of cluster headache are characteristic, and readily recognised by those familiar with the disorder. The brief, elegant description of the late Sir Charles Symonds[2] is often quoted in relation to the disorder:

> '...paroxysms of headache, that is to say, pain of sudden onset and transitory duration, which occurs in bouts lasting as a rule for several weeks with long periods of perfect freedom. In the paroxysm the pain is felt mainly in the supraorbital region or in and behind the eye, though it may spread beyond this region. It is, however, strictly unilateral. It is of agonising severity but very rarely lasts longer than two hours and often less. During a bout there is usually at least one paroxysm in each twenty-four hours: there may be more.'

However the condition was known long before Symonds' account.

Cluster headache, or migrainous neuralgia as it is commonly called in the British literature, affects males three or four times as often as females. It comprises attacks of unilateral pain usually in the forehead and temple but occasionally in the malar region. The pain usually develops rapidly, is almost always severe, sometimes throbbing in character, and lasts between a half hour and 3 hours in most instances. During attacks there is often ipsilateral conjunctival injection, tear production, nasal stuffiness or nasal discharge, and sometimes additional manifestations of an ipsilateral Horner's syndrome (ptosis and miosis).

Individual headache attacks are reasonably stereotyped, but the remarkable thing about the disorders is its time course. The attacks occur in clusters, each cluster lasting a period of several weeks to several months. During a cluster individual attacks usually occur several times a day and, particularly in the earlier weeks of a cluster, occur with an almost clockwork regularity at certain hours of the day and night. Once a cluster ceases (and clusters cease spontaneously) the sufferer remains free of attacks till the next cluster appears, often at the same season of the year, a year or more later. Consecutive clusters almost always affect the same side of the head in a given subject. Exceptionally, the attacks may be on different sides of the head in different clusters. During clusters, but not between clusters, alcohol intake characteristically provokes attacks within 1 or 2 hours. Ergotamine, taken orally or by injection two or three times a day for a few days, often seems to abort the attacks, particularly if used at any early stage in clusters.

Unlike the situation in migraine, a familial tendency to cluster headache is uncommon and there does not appear to be an increased incidence of family histories of migraine in cluster headache sufferers[3].

Cluster headache is a well-defined entity, clinically and diagnostically. The limits of the disorder are distinct, unlike those of migraine, though as mentioned earlier (Section 1.2) cluster headache variants are known, for example, chronic cluster headache and chronic paroxysmal hemicrania[4].

10.2 ALTERED FUNCTION AT A PHYSIOLOGICAL LEVEL

10.2.1 Individual attacks

10.2.1.1 Neurological manifestations

There are no prodromes, neurological or otherwise, to paroxysms of cluster headache. The sole neurological disturbance that may occur during attacks of cluster headache is Horner's syndrome. In theory this might arise from a lesion anywhere on a long circuitous neural loop from the hypothalamus via the brain stem and cervical cord to the cervical sympathetic trunk and the sympathetic plexuses around the internal carotid and ophthalmic arteries. However, observations during cluster headache attacks have shown that facial sweating may not be lost when the other manifestations of Horner's syndrome occur in the headache attacks. This suggests that the sympathetic paresis arises beyond the common carotid at the level of the internal carotid or ophthalmic artery. It has been suggested that an acute distension of the intracranial segment of the internal carotid artery might stretch the perivascular sympathetic plexus at this site to produce a temporary Horner's syndrome[5]. Ekbom and Greitz[6] described the findings of carotid angiography carried out in one subject during a cluster headache attack in which Horner's syndrome was present, without loss of facial sweating. There was a localised narrowing of the internal carotid artery just inside the skull, with considerable dilatation of the ophthalmic artery. Later, when the attack was subsiding, the area of carotid arterial narrowing had extended proximally into the carotid canal. With the use of thermography Wood and Friedman[7] noted persistent cool spots in the supraorbital region on the affected side in two-thirds of a series of 105 cases of cluster headache. The spots did not change during headache attacks. Kudrow[8], using thermographic and Doppler flow measurements, also found evidence of decreased ipsilateral frontal and supraorbital blood flow during cluster attacks and, to a lesser extent, between attacks. He interpreted this result as suggesting decreased internal carotid flow during clusters (the supraorbital artery is an internal carotid branch). Measurements of cerebral blood flow during cluster headache attacks have yielded somewhat contradictory results. Sakai *et al.*[9] and Sakai and Meyer[10] found increased flow, which they thought might be a post-ischaemic reaction. However Henry *et al.*[11] reported no change in flow in three subjects studied during attacks, and Nelson *et al.*[12] found decreased flow in three of the four subjects they investigated during attacks, and increased flow in the other subject. Thus the majority of the available evidence from the various sources favours decreased internal carotid flow during attacks of cluster headache. If the evidence of internal carotid artery narrowing and decreased cerebral blood flow during cluster headache attacks proves generally applicable, the idea of internal carotid artery distension causing sympathetic paresis becomes untenable, though ophthalmic artery distension might remain a possible cause for sympathetic injury. Could the basis for the sympathetic paresis be perivascular oedema and ischaemia[13]? There is no direct evidence of this. Any decreased internal carotid flow in cluster headache attacks is insufficient to disturb hemisphere function clinically. Much more severe decreases in internal carotid flow in other circumstances do not cause Horner's syndrome. Could it even be that the primary event in the attacks is unilateral sympathetic overactivity, which causes internal carotid artery spasm, with this then causing perivascular sympathetic ischaemic injury? Ekbom and Greitz[6] rejected the possibility of internal carotid artery spasm in the carotid canal, arguing that spasm at this site would be unlikely because it would produce a local vacuum within the bony walls of the canal.

10.2.1.2 Headache

The headache of migrainous neuralgia usually occurs in an area of the head that often corresponds tolerably well with the territory of supply of the ophthalmic division of the trigeminal nerve. This area of pain is also the area perfused for the most part by the superficial temporal artery. This artery may become distended and tender during attacks, and the character of the pain sometimes involves a pulsatile element. Compression of the superficial temporal artery may relieve the pain in the temple, though the compression may increase the pain in the eye; carotid compression in the neck relieves the ocular pain[14]. However, in occasional cluster headache sufferers, attacks occur in infraorbital nerve or maxillary division territory, areas whose blood supply is from the maxillary branches of the external carotid. Two hypotheses suggest themselves as explanations for these clinical observations concerning the pain of cluster headache. In one hypothesis, pain in the ophthalmic division territory or in maxillary division territory might be caused by temporary injury to these nerves in the cavernous sinus region (as suggested by Edmeads[13]). Whether internal carotid artery segmental spasm is a sufficient explanation for this postulated nerve injury seems very doubtful. Internal carotid distension at this level would be a more a more adequate explanation, and could also account for the sometimes pulsatile character of the pain. However, the evidence is against such dilatation occurring, as was pointed out above. The second line of hypothesis is that the pain is due to external carotid or supraorbital arterial dilatation, perhaps plus the local release of pain potentiating chemicals as is postulated to occur in migraine. The arterial dilatation may be a reactive change following ischaemia in internal carotid territory. The second hypothesis seems the more adequate, not because there is particularly strong evidence for it, but because there is some precedent for it in relation to migraine, and because the evidence runs against its alternative.

10.2.1.3 Associated features

The excess unilateral tear production and nasal congestion of cluster headache are not compatible with consequences of cervical sympathetic paralysis. It has been pointed out that excess parasympathetic activity conveyed via the greater superficial petrosal nerve could mediate the increased tear production and nasal stuffiness of cluster headache attacks[15]. It seems doubtful that dysfunction of the greater superficial petrosal nerve could mediate the pain of the disorder, since section of the nerve seems to have been abandoned as a surgical remedy for the condition.

10.2.2 Time pattern of the disorder

In general terms, one may suspect that activity of some biological clock mechanism is responsible for the highly characteristic time pattern of cluster headache attacks. Yet it must be a clock mechanism capable of accurate time-keeping over 24 hour time periods and also over time spans of several years (bearing in mind the seasonal occurrence of clusters). Admittedly the time-keeping mechanism might be 'set' repeatedly by cues from the environment, with its regular cycles, but there is no other disorder in all medicine in which a disturbance of bodily function occurs so consistently with such precise timing.

Biological 'clock' mechanisms in man are thought to reside in the hypothalamus, in particular in the suprachiasmatic nucleus, a structure which relays light-produced nerve impulses from the retina to the pineal (Section 8.2.4) and to other hypothalamic structures. The basis on which these hypothalamic mechanisms could be incriminated in cluster headache is inferential only. There is no direct evidence that they play any role. Whether the postulated hypothalamic processes merely set the timing for attacks initiated by other mechanisms, or whether these processes actually initiate the attacks, and initiate the clusters of attacks, is, in the present state of knowledge, entirely a matter for speculation.

The tendency of clusters to have a seasonal occurrence in a given individual might raise the question of allergy to some substance which occurs in the environment at particular times of the year. No such substance appears to have been traced in persons with cluster headache.

10.3 BIOCHEMICAL MECHANISMS UNDERLYING CLUSTER HEADACHE

10.3.1 Histamine

The biology of histamine, and its possible role in migraine pathogenesis, were discussed in Section 3.4. Interest in histamine in cluster headache began with Horton who termed the condition 'histaminic cephalgia' and reviewed his own considerable experience of the disorder in 1956[16]. He had observed that *during*, but not *between* clusters, a single subcutaneous injection of histamine was capable of activating cluster headache attacks. Horton's advocacy for the role of histamine in the condition tended to fall on deaf ears, possibly because he appeared to have seen so many more cases of histaminic cephalgia than the numbers of cases neurologists elsewhere recognised as having cluster headache (or migrainous neuralgia). However Anthony and Lance[17,18] found that plasma histamine levels rose during and remained elevated after cluster headache attacks in 19 out of 21 subjects. In an expanded group of subjects Anthony *et al.*[19] showed that mean plasma histamine levels before, during and after attacks were respectively 66.8, 76.7 and 63.1 ng/ml. The histamine levels rose in 45 of the 49 subjects they studied. Medina *et al.*[20] also found increased histamine levels in platelet-rich plasma from six subjects during cluster headache attacks. The histamine levels were higher in the external jugular blood from the side contralateral to the headache. The source of the histamine may be the increased numbers of mast cells that appear in attacks around the superficial temporal artery on the affected side[21] but also on the clinically unaffected side[22]. Sjaastad and Sjaastad[23] had earlier found increased urinary histamine excretion during cluster headache attacks in four out of eight subjects. The interpretation of this latter result is somewhat uncertain since urine pH was not measured and the possibility that the increased excretion might be due to diuresis was not considered. Sjaastad and Dale[24] mentioned that urine histamine excretion was increased in one of two cases of the rare and then new entity of chronic paroxysmal hemicrania. This disorder appears to be a cluster headache variant.

Kudrow[25] and Manzoni *et al.*[26] noted a statistically significant increase in peptic ulcer disease in cluster headache sufferers. This would be compatible with the effects of gastric hyperactivity from excess circulating histamine. Such hyperchlorhydria is known to occur in cluster headache[27]. Of course, other explanations for the gastro-intestinal dysfunction are possible.

Hardebo *et al.*[28] found a greater dilatational response to histamine *in vitro* in superficial temporal artery segments removed at biopsy from the affected side of cases of chronic cluster headache, as compared with the arteries from cases of classical cluster headache. This finding is difficult to interpret, as the biopsies had been done while the subjects were receiving drug therapy.

10.3.2 Serotonin

Anthony *et al.*[19] stated that there is no consistent alteration in whole plasma serotonin levels during cluster headache. In an earlier study in a smaller series of patients Anthony and Lance[17] had noted increased plasma serotonin levels in 19 cluster attacks, but decreased levels in eight and unchanged levels in two. Medina *et al.*[20] reported increased platelet serotonin concentrations at the onset of cluster attacks. Swade *et al.*[29] described a decreased V_{max} for platelet serotonin uptake during attacks of cluster headache in ten subjects. Salmon *et al.*[30] encountered increased levels of the serotonin precursor tryptophan in cerebrospinal fluid during cluster headache attacks. The significance of this finding is unclear.

10.3.3 Monoamine oxidase

Bussone *et al.*[31] noted reduced levels of platelet monoamine oxidase activity in seven cluster headache sufferers. The enzyme activity was less than that in the platelets of eight migraineurs, but the enzyme activity levels in these persons were also reduced, compared with normal control subjects. In view of the conflicting information that has emerged concerning platelet monoamine oxidase activity in migraine it may be premature to try to interpret these findings in cluster headache until more data become available.

10.3.4 Endogenous opioids

Anselmi *et al.*[32] reported decreased levels of enkephalins and γ-endorphin in the cerebrospinal fluid of cases of cluster headache. Appenzeller *et al.*[33] found that increased plasma levels of β-endorphin developed during cluster headache attacks. The increase was attributed to stress and agitation.

10.3.5 Free fatty acids

Anthony[34] noted the presence of increased plasma levels of free fatty acids in eight out of twelve cluster headache attacks studied. The implication of this finding is uncertain.

10.3.6 Testosterone

Kudrow[35] noted reduced circulating plasma testosterone levels during clusters as compared with testosterone levels in the same subjects during remissions, and also testosterone levels in normal control subjects. This finding has been confirmed by Klimek[36] and Romiti *et al.*[37], though Nelson[38] noted no significant difference in plasma testosterone levels between patients with cluster headache and patients with migraine. It has been suggested that the reduced testosterone levels are due to altered hypothalamic and pituitary function during clusters.

10.3.7 Prolactin

Polleri *et al.*[39] employed mathematical techniques to analyse the time courses of plasma prolactin levels in cluster headache sufferers. They interpreted their data as suggesting that prolactin secretion increased during attacks, perhaps as a response to stress.

10.3.8 Acetylcholine

Kunkle[40] found raised levels of what was identified by bioassay as acetylcholine in the cerebrospinal fluid of four out of fourteen patients during cluster headache attacks. It seems unwise to draw any conclusion from this work until the matter is studied again by modern chemical methods, though the relative infrequency of the reported changes suggests that this might not be a very rewarding line of investigation.

10.3.9 Chemical precipitation of cluster headache attacks

At least three agents are known precipitants of cluster headache attacks. These agents are histamine, glyceryl trinitrate and ethyl alcohol. Only the latter is likely to affect the nervous system directly, whereas all three are vasodilators. Although it is often risky to argue from known mechanisms of drug action to pathogenesis of a disorder, the above considerations would suggest that vasodilatation may have a role in precipitating attacks of cluster headache.

10.3.10 Chemical relief of cluster headache attacks

Apart from analgesics, the chemical agents known to relieve the pain of cluster headache are ergotamine (preferably administered parenterally) and inhaled oxygen[41]. Both are vasoconstrictors. Neither is known to have any direct effect on the normal central nervous system. The fact that vasoconstrictors relieve the pain of cluster headache suggests that vasodilatation contributes to, or causes, the pain.

10.4 EVALUATION OF THE MECHANISMS OF CLUSTER HEADACHE

10.4.1 Pain

The evidence, such as it is, appears to favour local scalp or facial vasodilatation as the mechanism of pain production in cluster headache attacks. Perivascular production of pain-causing chemicals may be involved, but experimental evidence of this is lacking as yet. The evidence appears to be against a cranial nerve basis for the pain origin, in that no suitable causative lesion has been demonstrated. The suggested pericarotid oedema in the cavernous sinus[13] seems scarcely adequate to injure trigeminal nerve branches. The possibility of a Sicuteri – Lance type hypothesis of unilateral locus coeruleus and mid-brain raphe disturbance causing cluster headache does not appear to have been raised in the literature. In cluster headache the pain usually remains unilateral in attacks and from cluster to cluster of attacks. Therefore one would not have to be bothered by the awkwardness of needing to invoke a shifting focus of brain stem disturbance to explain the features of the disorder, as would sometimes be necessary when the hypothesis is employed to explain migraine, with its more variably situated but still localised head pain.

Assuming that the pain of cluster headache is due to vasodilatation in the external carotid or supraorbital artery territories, and noting that the mechanisms of action of the chemicals provoking and relieving the pain (Sections 10.3.4 and 10.3.5) are consistent with this view, what is the biochemical mechanism of the pain? Increased circulating histamine levels of themselves do not provide a very adequate answer. Histamine levels appear to rise only after the headache has begun. Attempts to blockade both H_1 and H_2 type histamine receptors singly and simultaneously[19] have failed to prevent attacks of cluster headache. The serotonin changes that Medina *et al.*[20] have reported at an early stage in cluster headache attacks do not appear to have been confirmed by other workers. Further, these changes relate to serotonin in platelets. There is no information about serotonin free in plasma water. No circulating vasoactive substance should act only on the vessels of one side of the head. If a circulating chemical initiates cluster headache attacks, one would also have to invoke some local peculiarity of reaction of the relevant cranial blood vessels, or some abnormality of their neural control, to explain the pain localisation.

Thus we seem to lack sufficient evidence to explain the biochemical basis of the unilateral extracranial vasodilatation that appears to cause the pain of cluster headache. It seems very likely that some local factor is involved in the pain production, and if some circulating chemical agent is also involved the currently available evidence does not favour histamine, or serotonin. In some instances the local factor involved may be physical injury to tissue, however this is translated into molecular events. Manzoni *et al.*[26] have noted that if cluster headache develops subsequent to a head injury, the attacks often occur at the injury site.

10.4.2 Neurological manifestations

As discussed in Section 10.2.1, the explanation for the Horner's syndrome that occurs in some cluster headache attacks is not entirely satisfactory. On the whole it does seem likely that so localised a peripheral nervous system disturbance would have a local mechanical basis. Again, it seems desirable to invoke a local peculiarity of vascular and perivascular tissue chemistry to explain the Horner's syndrome, but the substances involved are unknown.

10.4.3 Associated features

The lateralised distribution of the altered tear production and the nasal congestion suggest a neural basis rather than a circulating biochemical basis for these manifestations. They could represent the consequences of parasympathetic overactivity in the territory of the greater superficial petrosal nerve. If so, the cause is obscure.

10.4.4 Time pattern of the disorder

As already discussed (Section 10.2.2), there appears to be no adequate explanation for the unique temporal pattern of cluster headache, either the individual attacks or the individual clusters. It is tempting to speculate that hypothalamic mechanisms are involved. The reduced plasma testosterone levels and altered prolactin secretion during clusters are consonant with this possibility, but there is no more direct proof of hypothalmic dysfunction.

In the present state of knowledge it is possible to explain at physiological level and in a moderately satisfactory way some of the cardinal manifestations of cluster headache. Current knowledge has not defined the biochemical factors responsible for initiating the clusters, or the individual attacks within clusters, or the biochemical factors which are responsible for the vasomotor changes and pain production in attacks. However, it seems likely that some of the relevant molecular changes will prove to have a localised anatomical distribution, and one might be tempted to speculate that release of chemicals into the circulation from hypothalamic 'time-keeping' mechanisms might determine the initiation of attacks, and of clusters, and thus be responsible for the highly characteristic time-pattern of the disorder.

References

1. Lance, J.W. and Anthony, M. (1973). Clinical and biochemical distinctions between migraine and migrainous neuralgia (cluster headache). In Cumings, J.N. (ed.). *Background to Migraine.* London: Heinemann, 116–121
2. Symonds, C.P. (1956). A particular variety of headache. *Brain,* **79,** 217–232
3. Sutherland, J.M. and Eadie, M.J. (1972). Cluster headache. *Research and Clinical Studies in Headache,* **3,** 92–125
4. Sjaastad, O., Russell, D., Saute, C. and Horven, I. (1982). Chronic paroxysmal hemicrania. VI. Precipitation of attacks. Further studies on the precipitation mechanism. *Cephalalgia,* **2,** 211–214
5. Kunkle, E.C. (1963). Headache mechanisms with particular reference to migraine. *Neurology,* **13,** 1–6
6. Ekbom, K. and Greitz, T. (1970). Carotid angiography in cluster headache. *Acta Radiologica. Diagnosis,* **20,** 177–186
7. Wood, E.H. and Friedman, A.P. (1974). Thermography in cluster headache. *Archives de Neurobiologica,* **37,** 85–93
8. Kudrow, L. (1979). Thermographic and Doppler flow asymmetry in cluster headache. *Headache,* **19,** 204–208
9. Sakai, F., Meyer, J.S., Ishihara, N., Naritomi, H. and Deshmukh, V.D. (1977). Noninvasive ^{133}Xe inhalation measurements of regional cerebral blood flow in migraine and related headaches. *Acta Neurologica Scandinavica, Suppl,* **56,** 196–197
10. Sakai, F. and Meyer, J.S. (1978). Regional cerebral hemodynamics during migraine and cluster headache measured by the ^{133}Xe inhalation method. *Headache,* **18,** 122–132
11. Henry, P.Y., Vernhiet, J., Orgogozo, J.M. and Caille, J.M. (1978). Cerebral blood flow in migraine and cluster headache. *Research and Clinical Studies in Headache,* **6,** 81–88
12. Nelson, R.F., Du Boulay, G.H., Marshall, J., Ross Russell, R.W., Symon, L. and Zilkha, E. (1980). Cerebral blood flow studies in patients with cluster headache. *Headache,* **20,** 184–189
13. Edmeads, J. (1979). Vascular headaches and the cranial circulation – another look. *Headache,* **19,** 127–131
14. Ekbom, K. (1975). Some observation on pain in cluster headache. *Headache,* **14,** 219–225
15. Gardner, W.J., Stowell, A. and Dutlinger, R. (1947). Resection of the greater superficial petrosal nerve in the treatment of unilateral headache. *Journal of Neurosurgery,* **41,** 105–114
16. Horton, B.T. (1956). Histaminic cephalgia. Differential diagnosis and treatment: 1176 patients 1937–1955. *Proceedings of the Staff Meetings of the Mayo Clinic,* **31,** 325–333
17. Anthony, M. and Lance, J.W. (1971). Whole blood histamine and plasma serotonin in cluster headache. *Proceedings of the Australian Association of Neurologists,* **8,** 43–46
18. Anthony, M. and Lance, J.W. (1971). Histamine and serotonin in cluster headache. *Archives of Neurology,* **25,** 225–231
19. Anthony, M., Lance, J.W. and Lord, G. (1978). Migrainous neuralgia – blood histamine levels and clinical response to H_1 and H_2 receptor blockade. In Greene, R. (ed.). *Current Concepts in Migraine Research.* New York: Raven Press, 149–158
20. Medina, J.L., Diamond, S. and Fareed, J. (1979). The nature of cluster headache. *Headache,* **19,** 309–322
21. Prusiński, A. and Liberski, P.O. (1979). Is the cluster headache local mastocytic diathesis? *Headache,* **19,** 102
22. Liberski, P.P. and Prusiński, A. (1982). Further observations on the mast cells over the painful region in cluster headache patients. *Headache,* **22,** 115–117
23. Sjaastad, O. and Sjaastad, O.V. (1970). The histaminuria in vascular headache. *Acta Neurologica Scandinavica,* **46,** 311–342
24. Sjaastad, O. and Dale, I. (1976). A new (?) clinical entity 'chronic paroxysmal hemicrania', 2. *Acta Neurologica Scandinavica,* **54,** 140–159
25. Kudrow, L. (1976). Prevalence of migraine, peptic ulcer, coronary heart disorder and hypertension in cluster headache. *Headache,* **16,** 66–69
26. Manzoni, G.C., Terzano, M.G., Bono, G., Micieli, G., Martucci, N. and Nappi, G. (1983). Cluster headache – clinical findings in 180 patients. *Cephalalgia,* **3,** 21–30

27. Horton, B.T. (1943). Histaminic cephalgia resulting in production of acute duodenal ulcers. *Journal of the American Medical Association,* **122,** 59–62
28. Hardebo, J.E., Krabbe, A.A. and Gjerris, F. (1980). Enhanced dilatory response to histamine in large extracranial vessels in chronic cluster headache. *Headache,* **20,** 316–320
29. Swade, C.C., Carroll, J.D. and Coppen, A. (1981). Platelet 5-hydroxytryptamine accumulation in migrainous neuralgia. In Rose, F.C. and Zilkha, K.J. (eds.). *Progress in Migraine Research. 1.* London: Pitman, 89–92
30. Salmon, S., Bonciani, M., Fanciullacci, M., Marianelli, L., Michelacci, S. and Sicuteri, F. (1982). A putative 5-HT control feedback in migraine and cluster headache attacks. In Critchley, M., Friedman, A.P., Gorini, S. and Sicuteri, F. (eds.). *Headache – Physiopathological and Clinical Concepts. Advances in Neurology,* **33,** 265–274
31. Bussone, G., Giovannini, P., Boiardi, A. and Boeri, R. (1977). A study of the activity of platelet monoamine oxidase in patients with migraine headaches or with 'cluster' headaches. *European Neurology,* **15,** 157–162
32. Anselmi, B., Baldi, E., Casacci, F. and Salmon, S. (1980). Endogenous opioids in cerebrospinal fluid and blood in idiopathic headache sufferers. *Headache,* **20,** 294–299
33. Appenzeller, O., Atkinson, R.A. and Standefer, J.C. (1981). Serum β-endorphin in cluster headache and common migraine. In Rose, F.C. and Zilkha, K.J. (eds.). *Progress in Migraine Research. 1.* London: Pitman, 106–109
34. *Anthony, M. (1976).* Plasma free fatty acids and prostaglandin E_1 in migraine and stress. *Headache,* **16,** 58–63
35. Kudrow, L. (1976). Plasma testosterone levels in cluster headache. Preliminary results. *Headache,* **16,** 28–31
36. Klimek, A. (1982). Plasma testosterone levels in patients with cluster headache. *Headache,* **22,** 162–164
37. Romiti, A., Martelletti, P., Giallo, M.F. and Giacovazzo, M. (1983). Low plasma testosterone levels in cluster headache. *Cephalalgia,* **3,** 41–44
38. Nelson, R.F.(1978). Testosterone level in cluster and non-cluster migrainous headache patients. *Headache,* **18,** 265–267
39. Polleri, A., Nappi, G., Murialdo, G., Bono, G., Martignoni, E. and Savoldi, F. (1982). Changes in the 24- hour prolactin pattern in cluster headache. *Cephalalgia,* **2,** 1–7
40. Kunkle, E.C. (1959). Acetylcholine in the mechanism of headache of the migraine type. *Archives of Neurology and Psychiatry,* **84,** 135–141
41. Kudrow, L. (1981). Response of cluster headache attacks to oxygen inhalation. *Headache,* **21,** 1–4

Index